THE POCKET

Protein Counter

Boost your protein intake for peak performance and fitness! In this handy pocket-size companion to *The Protein Counter* you have the perfect guide when food shopping, dining out, traveling, or camping. Take it with you wherever you go! *THE POCKET PROTEIN COUNTER* makes it easy to choose the optimum foods for life on the fast track!

———————

ANNETTE B. NATOW, Ph.D., R.D., and JO-ANN HESLIN, M.A., R.D., are the authors of twenty-one books on nutrition. Both are former faculty members of Adelphi University and the State University of New York, Downstate Medical Center. They are editors of the *Journal of Nutrition for the Elderly,* serve as editorial board members for the *Environmental Nutrition Newsletter,* and are frequent contributors to magazines and journals.

Books by Annette B. Natow and Jo-Ann Heslin

The Antioxidant Vitamin Counter
The Calorie Counter
The Cholesterol Counter (Fourth Edition)
The Diabetes Carbohydrate and Calorie Counter
The Fast-Food Nutrition Counter
The Fat Attack Plan
The Fat Counter (Third Edition)
The Iron Counter
Megadoses
No-Nonsense Nutrition for Kids
The Pocket Encyclopedia of Nutrition
The Pocket Fat Counter
The Pocket Protein Counter
The Pregnancy Nutrition Counter
The Protein Counter
The Sodium Counter
The Supermarket Nutrition Counter (Second Edition)

Published by POCKET BOOKS

THE POCKET
PROTEIN
COUNTER

ANNETTE B. NATOW, Ph.D., R.D.
and
JO-ANN HESLIN, M.A., R.D.

POCKET BOOKS
New York London Toronto Sydney Tokyo Singapore

An *Original* Publication of POCKET BOOKS

POCKET BOOKS, a division of Simon & Schuster Inc.
1230 Avenue of the Americas, New York, NY 10020

ISBN : 0-671-00380-1

First Pocket Books printing May 1997

10   9   8

POCKET and colophon are registered trademarks of Simon & Schuster Inc.

Cover design by Tom McKeven

Printed in the U.S.A.

"The fact that protein food is both a fuel and a building material makes its place in the diet confusing."

Mary Swartz Rose, Ph.D.
Feeding the Family
The Macmillan Company, 1919

To our families, who support us through
every project: Harry, Allen, Irene, Sarah,
Meryl, Laura, Marty, George, Emily, Steven,
Joe, Kristen and Karen

Acknowledgments

Without the tireless cooperation of Steven and Stephen, *The Pocket Protein Counter* would never have been completed. Our thanks to all the food manufacturers and processors who shared product information. A special thanks to our editor, Peter Wolverton, and our agent, Nancy Trichter.

Sources of Data

Values in this counter have been obtained from the Composition of Foods, United States Department of Agriculture, Agricultural Handbooks: No. 8–1, Dairy and Egg Products; No. 8–2, Spices and Herbs; No. 8–3, Baby Foods; No. 8–4, Fats and Oils; No. 8–5, Poultry Products; No. 8–6, Soups, Sauces and Gravies; No. 8–7, Sausages and Luncheon Meats; No. 8–8, Breakfast Cereals; No. 8–9, Fruit and Fruit Juices; No. 8–10, Pork Products; No. 8–11, Vegetables and Vegetable Products; No. 8–12, Nut and Seed Products; No. 8–13, Beef Products; No. 8–14, Beverages; No. 8–15, Finfish and Shellfish Products; No. 8–16, Legumes and Legume Products; No. 8–17, Lamb, Veal and Game Products; No. 8–18, Baked Products; No. 8–19, Snacks and Sweets; No. 8–20, Cereal Grains and Pasta; No. 8–21, Fast Foods; Supplements 1989, 1990, 1991, 1992.

"Nutritive Value of Foods." United States Department of Agriculture, Home and Garden Bulletin No. 72.

J. Davies and J. Dickerson, *Nutrient Content of Food Portions.* Cambridge, UK: The Royal Society of Chemistry, 1991.

G. A. Leveille, M. E. Zabik, and K. J. Morgan, *Nutrients in Foods.* Cambridge, MA: The Nutrition Guild, 1983.

A. Moller, E. Saxholt, and B. E. Mikkelsen, *Food Composition Tables Amino-acids, Carbohydrates and Fatty Acids in Danish Foods.* 1991.

Souci, Fachman, and Kraut, *Food Composition and Nutrition Tables.* Stuttgart: Wissenschaftliche Veriagsgesellschaft MbH, 1989.

Information from food labels, manufacturers and processors: The values are based on research conducted through the first half of 1996. Manufacturers' ingredients are subject to change, so current values may vary from those listed in the book. If the serving size on the package label is different from that listed in this counter, use the nutrition information provided as a guide. If the nutrition information listed in the Nutrition Facts panel is different from the information in this counter, assume that the product has been recently reformulated.

Introduction

Every day your body loses millions of cells. They are used up, worn out, rubbed off and even cut off like your beard or fingernails. You need protein to replace these cells.

Except for water, there is more protein in your body than anything else. A 143-pound man has over 25 pounds of protein!

Protein is found in every cell, tissue and substance in the body except for urine and bile. Our bodies contain many thousands of specific proteins, each one different and designed to do its special job. Bones, teeth, muscles, enzymes, skin and blood all contain protein. Active tissues, like muscles and glands, are high in protein, whereas less active tissue, like fat, has less.

When you don't get enough protein to replace lost cells and maintain normal functions, your body will cannibalize its own tissues and begin to waste away. That's why it is so important to get enough protein. But you should realize, excess protein is of no benefit to the body. It is not stored. It is simply used up for energy or converted to fat and then stored. Converting the protein to energy or fat makes the liver and kidneys work overtime as they process the extra protein and get rid of the leftover waste.

Protein is very important because it is

- Necessary for life.
- Necessary for growth.
- Part of every cell in your body.
- Needed to replace worn-out cells.
- Necessary to repair damaged tissue.
- A major part of the immune system.
- A major part of every enzyme.
- A source of energy.

You get protein from the food you eat. Foods like meat, milk, beans, vegetables and grains contain protein, which in turn supplies *amino acids*. Your body uses amino acids as the building blocks to make the special proteins it needs. All body proteins are made from about 20 different amino acids. These amino acids combine in different ways to make distinct kinds of protein in the same way that different letters of the alphabet combine to form many different words.

Amino Acids Are Very Special

Almost all foods contain protein, some more, some less. Fruits have little protein compared to meat, milk, cheese, beans, grains and vegetables. When you eat different foods, you get varying amounts of protein and varying amounts of the different amino acids they contain. Of the twenty different amino acids found in food, nine are essential. *These nine must be obtained directly in the food you eat.* The remaining eleven can be made in the body. This is one of the reasons why it is so important to eat a variety of protein foods. It guarantees you'll get all the different amino acids you need. For example, beans may be short in one of the essential amino acids, while rice and other grains have plenty of it. When you eat beans and rice together or even separately during the day, their amino acids pool together so that your body has a supply of all the amino acids needed to build its cells.

Necessary Nitrogen

Protein is different from the other energy sources we eat, like carbohydrate and fat, because it contains nitrogen. The need for protein is really a need for nitrogen. We lose nitrogen each day in urine, feces, skin, hair, nails, perspiration and other secretions. The nitrogen is replaced in the protein we eat.

YOUR DAILY PROTEIN FACTOR

Helps to Determine How Much Protein You Need Each Day

Age or Condition	Grams Protein per Kilogram of Target Weight
Teens	
Males	.9
Females	.8
Adults	.8
Mature adults	1.0
Recreational athlete	.8 to 1.0
Endurance athlete	1.2 to 1.8
Strength exercise	1.7 to 1.8
Strenuous exercise*	1.8 to 2.0
Mature athletes	1.0 to 1.5
Infections, fractures, fever, surgery	1.0 to 1.4
Severe trauma	1.5 to 2.5
Pregnancy	1.3 to 1.5
Breastfeeding	
1st six months	.8 + 15 grams
2nd six months	.8 + 12 grams

*Daily exercise program of one hour or more
Adapted from: Recommended Dietary Allowances, 10th edition, 1989, National Academy of Sciences, National Academy Press, Washington, DC; P.W.R. Lemon, Is Increased Dietary Protein Necessary or Beneficial for Individuals with a Physically Active Lifestyle, *Nutrition Reviews,* 54(4, Part II):S169, 1996; G.A. Edwald, MD and C.R. McKenzie, MD, Eds., Manual of Medical Therapeutics, 28th Ed., Boston: Little Brown & Co., Pg. 31, 1995.

Figuring Your Daily Protein Requirement

1. **Determine your daily protein factor.**
   Check the chart "Your Daily Protein Factor" above to determine the category that is right for you.

Example: If you are a recreational athlete your protein factor is .8 to 1.0 grams of protein.

YOUR DAILY PROTEIN FACTOR IS: _____

2. Find your "best" or "target" weight.

Your protein requirement is based on your weight. Here is a simple way to determine your target weight.

Women
Give yourself 100 pounds for the first 5 feet of your height and add 5 pounds for each additional inch over 5 feet (or subtract 5 pounds for each inch under 5 feet).
Example: If you're 5 feet 6 inches tall:

   100 pounds (for the first 5 feet)
 +30 pounds (6 additional inches × 5 pounds each)

130 pounds Target weight

Men
Give yourself 106 pounds for the first 5 feet of your height and add 6 pounds for each additional inch over 5 feet.
Example: If you're 5 feet 9 inches tall:

   106 pounds (for the first 5 feet)
 +54 pounds (9 additional inches X 6 pounds each)

160 pounds Target weight

Add 10% for a large body frame; subtract 10% for a small body frame. Not sure of your frame size—a large shoe size is a good predictor of a large frame.

_____ pounds (for the first 5 feet)
+ _____ pounds (_____ additional inches
                    × _____ pounds each)
_____ pounds Target weight

YOUR TARGET WEIGHT: _____

3. **Convert your weight in pounds to kilograms.**
   To determine your weight in kilograms, divide your weight in pounds by 2.2.

   _____ your weight (or target weight) ÷ 2.2 = _____ kilograms

   YOUR WEIGHT IN KILOGRAMS: _____

4. **Setting your daily requirement for protein.**
   Multiply your protein factor (from Step #1) × your weight in kilograms (from Step #3).
   Example: If you are a recreational athlete weighing 75 kilograms, your daily protein factor would be 0.8 to 1.0.

   0.8 (protein factor) × 75 kilograms = 60 grams of protein/day
   1.0 (protein factor) × 75 kilograms = 75 grams of protein/day

   A recreational athlete weighing 75 kilograms should be eating a minimum of 60 to 75 grams of protein each day.

   _____ your protein factor × _____ kilograms of weight = grams
   protein/day

   YOUR DAILY PROTEIN REQUIREMENT IS _____ GRAMS

   Now that you know how many grams of protein your need each day, use *The Pocket Protein Counter* to select the best choices to meet your needs. If your situation changes, you become pregnant or perhaps you change your exercise program to a more vigorous schedule, simply use Steps 1 to 4 to recalculate your daily protein requirement.

   Whether you want to track your protein intake for the day or you'd like to set up a complete eating plan that includes protein, fat and carbohydrate, *The Pocket Protein Counter* is the best guide you can use.

   Eat well—Stay Active—Be Well!

Caution: If you are thinking about increasing your daily protein by going to a high-protein diet, be sure to check with your doctor. Many medical experts feel very high-protein diets are not for everyone. People with heart conditions or who are on medication for heart disease, high blood pressure or diabetes need medical supervision for a very high protein diet.

Using Your Pocket Protein Counter

This book lists the protein, carbohydrate, fat and calorie content of more than 1,800 foods. With *The Pocket Protein Counter* in your pocket, it's easy to choose good protein foods. Because of this book's size, you may not always find your favorite brands listed. You will find enough—a few typical brand names and nonbranded samples—to make a good estimate of the protein content of everything you eat.

All foods are listed alphabetically, A to Z. The nonbranded (generic) listings are first, followed by a brand-name list. Many meat and fish entries are given in 3-ounce portions. They are equal in size to a tape cassette or a deck of cards.

When you need a bigger reference—one with counts for more than 15,000 foods—go to *The Protein Counter*.

EQUIVALENT MEASURES

DRY

3 teaspoons	=	1 tablespoon
4 tablespoons	=	¼ cup
8 tablespoons	=	½ cup
12 tablespoons	=	¾ cup
16 tablespoons	=	1 cup
1000 milligrams	=	1 gram
28 grams	=	1 ounce
4 ounces	=	¼ pound
8 ounces	=	½ pound
12 ounces	=	¾ pound
16 ounces	=	1 pound

LIQUID

2 tablespoons	=	1 ounce
¼ cup	=	2 ounces
½ cup	=	4 ounces
¾ cup	=	6 ounces
1 cup	=	8 ounces
2 cups	=	1 pint
4 cups	=	1 quart

ABBREVIATIONS

avg	=	average	prep	=	prepared
diam	=	diameter	pt	=	pint
fl	=	fluid	qt	=	quart
frzn	=	frozen	reg	=	regular
g	=	gram	serv	=	serving
in	=	inch	sm	=	small
lb	=	pound	sq	=	square
lg	=	large	tbsp	=	tablespoon
med	=	medium	tr	=	trace
mg	=	milligram	tsp	=	teaspoon
oz	=	ounce	w/	=	with
pkg	=	package	w/o	=	without

NOTES

Protein, carbohydrate and fat values are given in grams (g).

A dash (—) indicates data not available.

Discrepancies in figures are due to rounding, product reformulation and reevaluation. Labeling law allows rounding of values. Most of the data are analysis data obtained directly from manufacturers, not from labels. In some cases, our values may not be exactly the same as label information because they have not been rounded.

FOOD	PORTION	CALS.	CARB.	FAT	PRO.
ALFALFA					
sprouts	1 tbsp	1	tr	tr	tr
ALLIGATOR					
tail cooked	3½ oz	143	1	3	29
ALMONDS					
almond butter w/ salt	1 tbsp	101	3	9	2
almond butter w/o salt	1 tbsp	101	3	10	2
almond meal	1 oz	116	8	5	11
dry roasted unblanched	1 oz	167	7	15	5
Planters					
Almonds	1 oz	170	5	15	6
ANCHOVY					
canned in oil	5	42	0	2	6
ANTELOPE					
roasted	3 oz	127	0	2	25
APPLE					
dried rings	10	155	42	tr	1
fresh apple	1	81	21	tr	tr
APPLE JUICE					
After The Fall					
Organic	1 bottle (10 oz)	110	28	0	0
Minute Maid					
Box	8.45 fl oz	120	29	0	0
APPLESAUCE					
sweetened	½ cup	97	25	tr	tr
unsweetened	½ cup	53	14	tr	tr
APRICOT JUICE					
nectar	1 cup	141	36	tr	1
APRICOTS					
dried halves	10	83	22	tr	1
fresh apricots	3	51	12	tr	1
ARTICHOKE					
boiled	1 med (4 oz)	60	13	tr	4
S&W					
Hearts Marinated	½ cup	225	6	26	2
ARUGULA					
raw	½ cup	2	tr	tr	tr

FOOD	PORTION	CALS.	CARB.	FAT	PRO.
ASPARAGUS					
cooked	4 spears	14	3	tr	2
AVOCADO					
avocado	1	324	15	31	4
BACON					
cooked	3 strips	109	tr	9	6
BACON SUBSTITUTES					
Bac-Os					
Pieces	2 tsp (5 g)	25	2	1	2
BAGEL					
cinnamon raisin	1 (3½ in)	194	39	1	7
egg	1 (3½ in)	197	38	2	8
plain	1 (3½ in)	195	38	1	8
poppy seed	1 (3½ in)	195	38	1	8
BAMBOO SHOOTS					
sliced	1 cup	25	4	1	2
BANANA					
banana	1	105	27	tr	1
banana chips	1 oz	147	17	10	1
BANANA JUICE					
Libby					
Nectar	1 can (11.5 fl oz)	190	47	0	0
BASS					
striped baked	3 oz	105	0	3	19
BEAN SPROUTS					
La Choy					
	⅔ cup	8	1	tr	1
BEANS					
baked beans plain	½ cup	118	26	1	6
baked beans vegetarian	½ cup	118	26	1	6
refried beans	½ cup	134	23	1	8
Green Giant					
Three Bean Salad	½ cup	70	18	tr	2
BEEF					
brisket lean & fat trim ¼ in braised	3 oz	309	0	24	21
chuck pot roast lean & fat trim ¼ in braised	3 oz	282	0	20	23
corned beef brisket cooked	3 oz	213	tr	16	15

FOOD	PORTION	CALS.	CARB.	FAT	PRO.
corned beef canned	3 oz	85	0	5	10
eye of round lean & fat trim 0 in Choice roasted	3 oz	153	0	5	24
filet lean & fat trim ¼ in Choice broiled	3 oz	259	0	19	21
flank lean & fat trim 0 in broiled	3 oz	192	0	11	22
ground extra lean broiled medium	3 oz	217	0	14	22
ground extra lean fried medium	3 oz	216	0	14	21
ground regular broiled medium	3 oz	246	0	18	20
porterhouse steak lean & fat trim ¼ in Choice broiled	3 oz	260	0	19	21
roast beef medium	2 oz	70	0	2	12
shortribs lean & fat Choice braised	3 oz	400	0	36	18
standing rib lean & fat trim ¼ in Choice roasted	3 oz	320	0	27	19
t-bone steak lean & fat trim ¼ in Choice broiled	3 oz	253	0	18	21
Hormel					
Pillow Pack Dried Beef	10 slices (1 oz)	45	1	1	8
BEEF DISHES					
corned beef hash canned	3 oz	155	9	10	10
irish stew	1 cup (7 oz)	280	10	16	23
kebab indian	1 (5.4 oz)	553	2	40	47
koftas	5	280	3	22	18
roast beef sandwich plain	1	346	33	14	22
roast beef submarine sandwich w/ tomato lettuce & mayonnaise	1	411	44	13	29
samosa	2 (4 oz)	652	20	62	6
stroganoff	¾ cup	260	43	19	14
swiss steak	4.6 oz	214	10	9	23
Casbah					
Gyro as prep	1 patty (2 oz)	145	12	5	2
Dinty Moore					
Microwave Cup Beef Stew	1 cup (7.5 oz)	190	15	10	11
Hamburger Helper					
Nacho Cheese as prep	1 cup	360	35	15	21
Hot Pocket					
Stuffed Sandwich Beef & Cheddar	1 (4.5 oz)	360	36	18	14

FOOD	PORTION	CALS.	CARB.	FAT	PRO.
Lean Pockets					
Stuffed Sandwich Beef & Broccoli	1 (4.5 oz)	250	37	7	9
Manwich					
Sloppy Joe as prep	1 sandwich	310	31	13	17
BEER AND ALE					
ale brown	10 oz	77	8	0	1
ale pale	10 oz	88	12	0	1
beer light	12 oz can	100	5	0	tr
beer regular	12 oz can	146	13	0	1
BEET JUICE					
juice	3½ oz	36	8	0	1
BEETS					
harvard	½ cup	89	22	tr	1
pickled	½ cup	75	19	tr	1
sliced cooked	½ cup	27	6	tr	1
BISCUIT					
buttermilk	1	127	17	6	2
plain	1 (35 g)	276	13	34	4
w/ egg	1	315	24	20	11
w/ egg & bacon	1	457	29	31	17
w/ egg & sausage	1	582	41	39	19
w/ egg & steak	1	474	37	28	18
w/ egg cheese & bacon	1	477	33	31	16
w/ ham	1	387	44	18	13
w/ sausage	1	485	40	32	12
BLACK BEANS					
cooked	1 cup	227	41	1	15
Mahatma					
Black Beans & Rice	1 cup	200	39	2	8
BLACKBERRIES					
blackberries	½ cup	37	9	tr	1
BLACKEYE PEAS					
cooked	1 cup	198	36	1	13
BLINTZE					
cheese	2	186	18	6	13
BLUEBERRIES					
blueberries	1 cup	82	20	1	1

FOOD	PORTION	CALS.	CARB.	FAT	PRO.
Sonoma					
Dried	¼ cup (1.3 oz)	140	33	0	1
BLUEFISH					
fresh baked	3 oz	135	0	5	22
BOK CHOY					
Dole					
Shredded	½ cup	5	1	tr	1
BOYSENBERRY JUICE					
Smucker's					
Juice	8 oz	120	30	0	0
BRAINS					
beef pan-fried	3 oz	167	0	13	11
BRAN					
oat cooked	½ cup	44	13	tr	4
Kretschmer					
Toasted Wheat Bran	⅓ cup	57	15	2	6
BRAZIL NUTS					
dried unblanched	1 oz	186	4	19	4
BREAD					
chapatis as prep w/ fat	1 (2½ oz)	230	34	9	6
cornstick	1 (1.3 oz)	101	13	4	2
cracked wheat	1 slice	65	12	1	2
focaccia rosemary	1 piece (3.5 oz)	251	40	7	6
focaccia tomato olive	1 piece (4.7 oz)	270	42	8	6
french	1 slice (1 oz)	78	15	1	3
irish soda bread	1 slice (2 oz)	174	34	3	4
italian	1 slice (1 oz)	81	15	1	3
oat bran	1 slice	71	12	1	3
oat bran reduced calorie	1 slice	46	10	1	2
papadums fried	2 (1.5 oz)	81	9	4	4
paratha	1 (4.4 oz)	403	54	18	10
pita	1 reg (2 oz)	165	33	1	5
pita	1 sm (1 oz)	78	16	tr	3
protein	1 slice	47	8	tr	2
pumpernickel	1 slice	80	15	1	3
raisin	1 slice	71	14	1	2
rye	1 slice	83	16	1	3

FOOD	PORTION	CALS.	CARB.	FAT	PRO.
rye reduced calorie	1 slice	47	9	1	2
seven grain	1 slice	65	12	1	3
sourdough	1 slice (1 oz)	78	15	1	3
wheat berry	1 slice	65	12	1	2
white	1 slice	67	12	1	2
white reduced calorie	1 slice	48	10	1	2
whole wheat	1 slice	70	13	1	3
B&M					
Brown Bread	½ in slice (⅙ oz)	92	21	0	2
Damascus Bakeries					
Mountain Shepherd Lahvash	⅓ loaf (2 oz)	135	28	0	5
Kineret					
Challah	⅛ loaf (2 oz)	150	25	4	5
Matthew's					
Sodium Free	1 slice	70	12	2	3
Monks' Bread					
Hi-Fibre	1 slice	50	13	1	3
Stefano's					
Stuffed Bread Broccoli & Cheese	½ bread (6 oz)	450	54	17	19
Tree Of Life					
100% Spelt	1 slice (1.8 oz)	130	22	3	4
Wonder					
Calcium Enriched	1 slice (1 oz)	70	12	1	3

BREADSTICKS

FOOD	PORTION	CALS.	CARB.	FAT	PRO.
Angonoa					
Garlic	6 (1 oz)	120	21	2	4
Whole Wheat Mini	14 (1 oz)	130	19	4	4
Lance					
Cheese	2	20	4	0	tr
Pillsbury					
Soft Bread Sticks	1	100	17	2	3
Stella D'Oro					
Regular	1	40	7	1	1

BREAKFAST BAR

FOOD	PORTION	CALS.	CARB.	FAT	PRO.
Carnation					
Chewy Chocolate Chip	1 (1.26 oz)	150	22	6	2
Chewy Peanut Butter Chocolate Chip	1 (1.26 oz)	140	21	5	3

FOOD	PORTION	CALS.	CARB.	FAT	PRO.
Glenny's					
Sunrise Bee Pollen	1 bar (1.5 oz)	190	22	8	5
Sunrise Ginseng	1 bar (1.5 oz)	160	24	7	1
Sunrise Spirulina	1 bar (1.5 oz)	140	21	5	3
Nutri-Grain					
Strawberry	1 (1.3 oz)	140	27	3	2
BREAKFAST DRINKS					
Carnation					
Instant Breakfast Creamy Milk Chocolate	1 pkg + skim milk (9 fl oz)	220	39	1	12
Instant Breakfast No Sugar Added Classic Chocolate	1 pkg + skim milk (9 fl oz)	160	24	2	12
Pillsbury					
Instant Breakfast Strawberry as prep w/ milk	1 serving	290	39	9	14
Instant Breakfast Vanilla as prep w/ whole milk	1 serving	300	41	9	14
BROCCOLI					
spears cooked	½ cup	25	5	tr	3
Birds Eye					
With Cheese Sauce	½ pkg	110	9	5	5
BROWNIE					
plain	1 lg (2 oz)	227	36	9	3
w/o nuts	1 (2 oz)	243	39	10	3
Little Debbie					
Fudge	1 pkg (2.1 oz)	270	39	13	2
BRUSSELS SPROUTS					
fresh	½ cup	30	7	tr	2
BUCKWHEAT					
Wolff's					
Kasha Medium cooked	¼ cup (1.6 oz)	170	35	2	64
BULGUR					
cooked	½ cup	76	17	tr	3
BUTTER					
stick	1 pat	36	tr	4	tr
whipped	1 pat	27	tr	3	tr

FOOD	PORTION	CALS.	CARB.	FAT	PRO.
BUTTER SUBSTITUTES					
Butter Buds					
Sprinkles	1 tsp (2 g)	5	2	0	0
BUTTERFISH					
baked	3 oz	159	0	9	19
CABBAGE					
coleslaw w/ dressing	½ cup	42	7	2	1
green raw shredded	½ cup (1.2 oz)	9	2	tr	1
red raw shredded	½ cup	10	2	tr	tr
stuffed cabbage	1 (6 oz)	373	18	22	25
sweet & sour red cabbage	4 oz	61	8	3	1
CAKE					
angelfood	¹/₁₂ cake (1 oz)	73	16	tr	2
chocolate w/ chocolate frosting	⅛ cake (2.2 oz)	235	35	11	3
coffeecake crumb topped cinnamon	1/9 cake (2.2 oz)	263	29	15	4
pound	¹/₁₀ cake (1 oz)	117	15	6	2
pound fat free	1 oz	80	17	tr	2
sponge	¹/₁₂ cake (1.3 oz)	110	23	1	2
strudel apple	1 piece (2½ oz)	195	29	8	2
tiramisu	1 piece (5.1 oz)	409	31	30	7
yellow w/ vanilla frosting	⅛ cake (2.2 oz)	239	38	9	2
Drake's					
Coffee Cake Small	1 (2 oz)	220	33	9	3
Devil Dog	1 (1.5 oz)	160	24	6	2
Entenmann's					
Cinnamon Buns	1 (2.1 oz)	230	31	10	4
Hostess					
Cup Cakes Chocolate	1 (1.6 oz)	170	28	5	2
Cup Cakes Chocolate Light	1 (1.4 oz)	120	26	2	2
Twinkies	1 (1.4 oz)	140	25	4	1
Kellogg's					
Pop-Tarts Brown Sugar Cinnamon	1 (1.8 oz)	220	32	9	3
Rice Krispies Treats	1 (0.8 oz)	90	18	2	1
Little Debbie					
Jelly Rolls	1 pkg (2.1 oz)	230	41	7	1
Sara Lee					
French Cheese	1 slice (2.9 oz)	250	23	16	4

FOOD	PORTION	CALS.	CARB.	FAT	PRO.
Sinbad					
Baklava	1 piece (2 oz)	337	44	20	5
Tastykake					
Kandy Kake Peanut Butter	1 (19 g)	90	11	4	2
Thomas'					
Date Nut Loaf	1 oz	90	18	2	1
Toast-R-Cakes					
Corn	1	120	19	4	2
Weight Watchers					
Chocolate Eclair	1 (2.1 oz)	120	19	4	2
CALZONE					
cheese	1 (12 oz)	1020	86	54	48
CANADIAN BACON					
Jones					
Slices	1	30	tr	1	3
CANDY					
candy corn	1 oz	105	27	0	tr
caramels	1 piece (8 g)	31	6	1	tr
carob bar	1 (3.1 oz)	453	42	28	11
dark chocolate	1 oz	150	16	10	1
gumdrops	10 sm (0.4 oz)	135	35	0	0
gumdrops	10 lg (3.8 oz)	420	108	0	0
hard candy	1 oz	106	28	0	0
jelly beans	10 sm (0.4 oz)	40	10	tr	0
lollipop	1 (6 g)	22	6	0	0
milk chocolate w/ almonds	1 bar (1.45 oz)	215	22	14	4
peanuts chocolate covered	10 (1.4 oz)	208	20	13	5
pretzels chocolate covered	1 (0.4 oz)	50	8	2	1
Godiva					
Truffle Amaretto Di Saronno	2 pieces (1.5 oz)	210	24	12	2
Good & Plenty					
Snacksize	3 boxes (1.5 oz)	140	34	0	1
Hershey					
Kisses	9 pieces (1.46 oz)	220	23	13	3
Joyva					
Halvah	1.5 oz	240	16	16	4
Lifesavers					
Roll Five Flavor	2 pieces (5 g)	20	5	0	0

FOOD	PORTION	CALS.	CARB.	FAT	PRO.
M&M's					
Peanut	1 pkg (1.7 oz)	250	30	13	5
Plain	1 pkg (1.7 oz)	230	34	10	2
Nestle					
Milk Chocolate	1 bar (1.45 oz)	220	23	13	4
Pearson					
Licorice	2 pieces (0.5 oz)	60	12	2	0
Pez					
Candy	1 roll (0.3 oz)	30	8	0	0
Raisinets					
Raisins	1 pkg (1.58 oz)	200	31	8	2
Reese's					
Peanut Butter Cups	1 (1.8 oz)	280	26	17	6
Starburst					
Original Fruits	8 pieces (1.4 oz)	160	33	3	0
Twizzlers					
Candy	4 pieces (1.4 oz)	130	30	1	1
York					
Peppermint Patty	1 (1.5 oz)	180	34	4	1
Peppermint Patty	1 snack size (0.5 oz)	57	11	1	tr

CANTALOUPE

cubed	1 cup	57	13	tr	1
half	½	94	22	1	2

CARP

fresh cooked	3 oz	138	0	6	19

CARROT JUICE

Hain					
Juice	6 fl oz	80	17	0	1

CARROTS

baby raw	1 (0.5 oz)	6	1	tr	tr
raw	1 (2.5 oz)	31	7	tr	1
raw shredded	½ cup	24	6	tr	1
slices cooked	½ cup	35	8	tr	1

CASABA

cubed	1 cup	45	11	tr	2

CASHEWS

cashew butter w/o salt	1 tbsp	94	4	8	3
dry roasted salted	1 oz	163	9	13	4

FOOD	PORTION	CALS.	CARB.	FAT	PRO.
CATFISH					
channel breaded & fried	3 oz	194	7	11	15
CAULIFLOWER					
broccoflower raw	½ cup (1.8 oz)	16	3	tr	1
flowerets cooked	3 (2 oz)	12	2	tr	1
flowerets raw	3 (2 oz)	14	3	tr	1
Birds Eye					
With Cheese Sauce	½ pkg	90	8	5	5
CAVIAR					
black granular	1 tbsp	40	1	3	4
red granular	1 tbsp	40	1	3	4
CELERY					
diced cooked	½ cup	13	3	tr	1
raw	1 stalk (1.3 oz)	6	1	tr	tr
CEREAL					
Arrowhead					
Amaranth Flakes	1 cup (1.2 oz)	130	25	2	4
Bear Mush	¼ cup (1.6 oz)	160	33	1	5
Kamut Flakes	1 cup (1.1 oz)	120	25	1	4
Cap'n Crunch					
Original	¾ cup	113	24	2	2
Chex					
Corn	1¼ cup (1 oz)	110	26	0	2
Erewhon					
Oatmeal Instant Apple Cinnamon	1.25 oz	145	25	3	4
Estee					
Raisin Bran	1 pkg (1 oz)	90	21	1	4
General Mills					
Cheerios	1¼ cup (1 oz)	110	20	2	4
Cocoa Puffs	1 cup (1 oz)	110	25	1	1
Kix	1½ cup (1 oz)	110	24	1	2
Total	1 cup (1 oz)	100	22	1	3
Wheaties	1 cup (1 oz)	100	23	1	3
Good Shepherd					
Spelt	1 oz	90	20	tr	4
Health Valley					
Fruit & Fitness	1 cup (2 oz)	220	37	4	9

FOOD	PORTION	CALS.	CARB.	FAT	PRO.
Kashi					
Cereal	2 oz	177	38	1	6
Kellogg's					
All-Bran	½ cup (1 oz)	80	22	1	4
Corn Flakes	1 cup (1 oz)	110	26	0	2
Frosted Flakes	¾ cup (1 oz)	120	28	0	1
Product 19	1 cup (1 oz)	110	25	0	3
Raisin Bran	1 cup (1.9 oz)	170	43	1	5
Rice Krispies	1¼ cup (1 oz)	110	26	0	2
Special K	1 cup (1 oz)	110	21	0	6
Maltex					
Cereal	1 oz	105	21	1	3
Maypo					
30 Second	1 oz	100	19	1	4
McCann's					
Irish Oatmeal	1 oz	110	20	2	5
Nabisco					
Cream Of Wheat Instant as prep	1 cup	120	25	0	3
Shredded Wheat Spoon Size	⅔ cup (1 oz)	90	23	1	3
Pillsbury					
Farina	⅔ cup	80	17	tr	2
Quaker					
Instant Grits White Hominy	1 pkg	79	18	tr	2
Oatmeal Instant	1 pkg (1.2 oz)	130	22	3	5
Oats Old Fashion	½ cup	150	27	3	5
Puffed Rice	1 cup	54	13	tr	1
Shredded Wheat	2 biscuits	132	32	1	4
Roman Meal					
Cream Of Rye	1.3 oz	111	20	1	5
Stone-Buhr					
7 Grain	⅓ cup (1.6 oz)	140	31	2	6
Weetabix					
Cereal	2 (1.3 oz)	142	31	1	4
Wheatena					
Cereal	⅓ cup (1.4 oz)	150	32	1	5

CHAMPAGNE

Andre

Cold Duck	1 fl oz	25	2	0	0

FOOD	PORTION	CALS.	CARB.	FAT	PRO.
Ballatore					
Spumante	1 fl oz	23	2	0	0
Eden Roc					
Extra Dry	1 fl oz	21	1	0	0
CHAYOTE					
fresh cooked	1 cup	38	8	1	1
CHEESE					
bel paese	3½ oz	391	0	30	25
blue	1 oz	100	1	8	6
brick	1 oz	105	1	8	7
brie	1 oz	95	tr	8	8
camembert	1 wedge (1.3 oz)	114	tr	9	8
cheddar	1 oz	114	tr	9	7
cheddar low fat	1 oz	49	1	2	9
colby	1 oz	112	1	9	7
colby low fat	1 oz	49	1	2	9
edam	1 oz	101	tr	8	7
feta	1 oz	75	1	6	4
fontina	1 oz	110	tr	9	7
gjetost	1 oz	132	12	8	3
goat soft	1 oz	76	tr	6	5
gouda	1 oz	101	1	8	7
gruyere	1 oz	117	tr	9	8
limburger	1 oz	93	tr	8	8
monterey	1 oz	106	tr	9	7
mozzarella	1 oz	80	1	6	6
mozzarella part skim	1 oz	72	1	5	7
muenster	1 oz	104	tr	9	7
parmesan grated	1 tbsp	23	tr	2	2
provolone	1 oz	100	1	8	7
queso anego	1 oz	106	1	9	6
queso asadero	1 oz	101	1	8	6
queso chichuahua	1 oz	106	2	8	6
ricotta	½ cup	216	4	16	14
ricotta part skim	½ cup	171	6	10	14
romano	1 oz	110	1	8	9
roquefort	1 oz	105	1	9	6
stilton blue	1.4 oz	164	0	14	9

FOOD	PORTION	CALS.	CARB.	FAT	PRO.
swiss	1 oz	107	1	8	8
whey cheese	3.5 oz	440	33	27	15
Alouette					
Garlic	2 tbsp (0.8 oz)	70	1	7	1
Alpine Lace					
Fat Free Singles	1 slice (0.66 oz)	25	tr	0	5
Cheez Whiz					
Spread	2 tbsp (1.2 oz)	90	2	7	5
Dorman's					
Lo-Chol Cheddar	1 oz	100	1	7	7
Friendship					
Farmer	2 tbsp (1 oz)	50	0	3	5
Hoop	2 tbsp (1 oz)	20	0	0	5
Frigo					
Asiago	1 oz	110	1	9	7
String	1 oz	80	1	5	7
Handi-Snacks					
Cheez'n Crackers	1 pkg (1.1 oz)	130	10	8	4
Kraft					
Cheese With Jalapeno Peppers	1 oz	60	2	7	5
Free Singles Swiss	1 slice (0.7 oz)	30	3	0	5
Havarti	1 oz	120	0	11	6
Lactaid					
American	3.5 oz	328	7	25	20
Laughing Cow					
Assorted Wedge	1 (1 oz)	70	1	6	4
Babybel	1 oz	90	0	7	7
Light N'Lively					
Singles 50% Less Fat American	0.7 oz	50	2	3	5
Polly-O					
Mozzarella Free	1 oz	35	tr	0	7
Ricotta Free	¼ cup	50	2	0	10
Roka					
Spread Blue	2 tbsp (1.1 oz)	80	2	7	3
Sargento					
Jarlsberg	1 slice (1.2 oz)	120	1	9	9
Smart Beat					
American	1 slice (0.6 oz)	35	2	2	4

FOOD	PORTION	CALS.	CARB.	FAT	PRO.
Tree Of Life					
Colby Organic Milk	1 oz	120	1	10	7
Swiss Raw Milk	1 oz	110	1	8	8
Velveeta					
Cheese	1 slice (0.7 oz)	60	2	5	4
Weight Watchers					
American Slices Yellow	2 slices (⅔ oz)	35	1	1	4
WisPride					
Port Wine Cup	2 tbsp (1.1 oz)	100	4	7	4
CHEESE DISHES					
cheese omelette as prep w/ 2 eggs	1 (6.8 oz)	519	tr	44	31
macaroni & cheese	6.3 oz	320	25	19	13
CHEESE SUBSTITUTES					
White Wave					
Soy A Melt Cheddar	1 oz	80	1	5	8
Soy A Melt Fat Free Mozzarella	1 oz	40	3	tr	7
Soy A Melt Jalapeno Jack	1 oz	80	1	5	8
CHERRIES					
fresh sweet	10	49	11	1	1
CHERRY JUICE					
After The Fall					
Black Cherry	1 can (12 oz)	170	42	0	0
CHESTNUTS					
roasted	1 cup	350	76	3	5
CHEWING GUM					
bubble gum	1 block (8 g)	27	8	0	0
stick	1 (3 g)	10	3	0	0
CHICKEN					
boneless breaded & fried w/ barbecue sauce	6 pieces (4.6 oz)	330	25	18	17
boneless breaded & fried w/ honey	6 pieces (4 oz)	339	27	18	17
boneless breaded & fried w/ mustard sauce	6 pieces (4.6 oz)	323	21	17	17
boneless breaded & fried w/ sweet & sour sauce	6 pieces (4.6 oz)	346	29	18	17
breast & wing breaded & fried	2 pieces (5.7 oz)	494	20	30	36
broiler/fryer breast w/ skin batter dipped & fried	½ breast (4.9 oz)	364	13	18	35

FOOD	PORTION	CALS.	CARB.	FAT	PRO.
broiler/fryer breast w/ skin roasted	½ breast (3.4 oz)	193	0	8	29
broiler/fryer breast w/ skin stewed	½ breast (3.9 oz)	202	0	8	30
broiler/fryer breast w/o skin roasted	½ breast (3 oz)	142	0	3	27
broiler/fryer drumstick w/ skin batter dipped & fried	1 (2.6 oz)	193	6	11	16
broiler/fryer drumstick w/ skin floured & fried	1 (1.7 oz)	120	1	7	13
broiler/fryer drumstick w/ skin roasted	1 (1.8 oz)	112	0	6	14
broiler/fryer drumstick w/ skin stewed	1 (2 oz)	116	0	6	14
broiler/fryer drumstick w/o skin fried	1 (1.5 oz)	82	0	3	12
broiler/fryer drumstick w/o skin roasted	1 (1.5 oz)	76	0	2	12
broiler/fryer drumstick w/o skin stewed	1 (1.6 oz)	78	0	3	13
broiler/fryer leg w/ skin batter dipped & fried	1 (5.5 oz)	431	14	26	34
broiler/fryer leg w/ skin floured & fried	1 (3.9 oz)	285	3	16	30
broiler/fryer leg w/ skin roasted	1 (4 oz)	265	0	15	30
broiler/fryer leg w/ skin stewed	1 (4.4 oz)	275	0	16	30
broiler/fryer leg w/o skin fried	1 (3.3 oz)	195	1	9	27
broiler/fryer leg w/o skin roasted	1 (3.3 oz)	182	0	8	26
broiler/fryer leg w/o skin stewed	1 (3.5 oz)	187	0	8	26
broiler/fryer neck w/ skin stewed	1 (1.3 oz)	94	0	7	7
broiler/fryer skin roasted	from ½ chicken (2 oz)	254	0	23	11
broiler/fryer thigh w/ skin batter dipped & fried	1 (3 oz)	238	8	14	19
broiler/fryer thigh w/ skin floured & fried	1 (2.2 oz)	162	2	9	17
broiler/fryer thigh w/ skin stewed	1 (2.4 oz)	158	0	10	16
broiler/fryer thigh w/o skin fried	1 (1.8 oz)	113	1	5	15
broiler/fryer thigh w/o skin roasted	1 (1.8 oz)	109	0	6	13
broiler/fryer thigh w/o skin stewed	1 (1.9 oz)	107	0	5	14
broiler/fryer w/ skin floured & fried	½ chicken (11 oz)	844	10	47	90
broiler/fryer w/ skin fried	½ chicken (16.4 oz)	1347	44	81	81

FOOD	PORTION	CALS.	CARB.	FAT	PRO.
broiler/fryer w/ skin roasted	½ chicken (10.5 oz)	715	0	41	82
broiler/fryer w/ skin stewed	½ chicken (11.7 oz)	730	0	42	82
broiler/fryer w/o skin roasted	1 cup (5 oz)	266	0	10	41
broiler/fryer w/o skin stewed	1 cup (5 oz)	248	0	9	38
broiler/fryer wing w/ skin batter dipped & fried	1 (1.7 oz)	159	5	11	10
broiler/fryer wing w/ skin floured & fried	1 (1.1 oz)	103	1	7	8
broiler/fryer wing w/ skin roasted	1 (1.2 oz)	99	0	7	9
broiler/fryer wing w/ skin stewed	1 (1.4 oz)	100	0	7	9
canned w/ broth	1 can (5 oz)	234	0	11	31
chicken spread canned	1 tbsp	25	1	2	2
cornish hen w/o skin & bone roasted	½ hen (2 oz)	72	0	2	13
cornish hen w/o skin & bone roasted	1 hen (3.8 oz)	144	0	4	25
cornish hen w/skin roasted	½ hen (4 oz)	296	0	21	25
cornish hen w/skin roasted	1 hen (8 oz)	595	0	42	51
drumstick breaded & fried	2 pieces (5.2 oz)	430	16	27	30
oven roasted breast of chicken	2 oz	60	0	1	11
thigh breaded & fried	2 pieces (5.2 oz)	430	16	27	30
Banquet					
Wings Hot & Spicy	4 pieces (5 oz)	230	5	16	15
Carl Buddig					
Sliced	1 oz	50	1	3	5
Empire					
Nuggets	5 (3 oz)	180	12	9	13
Healthy Choice					
Deli-Thin Smoked Breast	6 slices (2 oz)	60	1	2	11
Hebrew National					
Deli Thin Oven Roasted	1.8 oz	45	—	1	10
Hillshire					
Flavor Pack 90-99% Fat Free Smoked Breast	1 slice (0.75 oz)	20	tr	tr	4
Lunch 'N Munch Smoked Chicken/ Monterey/ Snickers	1 pkg (4.25 oz)	400	31	23	19
Oscar Mayer					
Deli-Thin Honey Glazed Breast	4 slices (1.8 oz)	60	2	1	10

FOOD	PORTION	CALS.	CARB.	FAT	PRO.
Oscar Mayer (CONT.)					
Lunchables Dessert Chocolate Pudding/Chicken/ Jack	1 pkg (6.2 oz)	370	33	18	19
Perdue					
Nuggets Cheese	1 (.67 oz)	54	3	4	3
Tyson					
Bologna	1 slice	44	4	1	2
Cordon Blue Mini	1	90	5	4	8
Wampler Longacre					
Ground raw	1 oz	50	0	4	4
Roll Sliced	1 slice (0.8 oz)	50	1	4	4
Weaver					
Croquettes	2 pieces	280	22	16	14
Rondelets Original	1 (3 oz)	190	13	10	13
Weight Watchers					
Roasted Ham	2 slices (¾ oz)	25	tr	1	4
CHICKEN DISHES					
chicken & dumplings	¾ cup	256	12	12	23
chicken & noodles	1 cup	365	26	18	22
chicken a la king	1 cup	470	12	34	27
chicken pie w/ top crust	1 slice (5.6 oz)	472	32	31	19
fillet sandwich plain	1	515	39	29	24
fillet sandwich w/ cheese lettuce mayonnaise & tomato	1	632	42	39	29
Hot Pocket					
Stuffed Sandwich Chicken & Cheddar With Broccoli	1 (4.5 oz)	300	37	12	12
Lean Pockets					
Stuffed Sandwich Chicken Fijita	1 (4.5 oz)	260	36	8	12
Skillet Chicken Helper					
Fettucine Alfredo as prep	⅕ pkg (7.5 oz)	270	29	8	21
Wampler Longacre					
Cacciatore	1 serv (4 oz)	118	5	3	14
Weight Watchers					
Chicken & Broccoli Pita	1 (5.4 oz)	190	19	5	15
White Castle					
Grilled Chicken Sandwich	2 (4 oz)	250	24	9	17
CHICKEN SUBSTITUTES					
Harvest Direct					
TVP Poultry Ground	3.5 oz	280	32	1	52

FOOD	PORTION	CALS.	CARB.	FAT	PRO.
LaLoma					
Fried Chicken w/ Gravy	2 piece (85 g)	140	4	10	9
White Wave					
Meatless Sandwich Slices	2 slices (1.6 oz)	80	8	0	12
Worthington					
Chick-ketts	½ cup (84 g)	160	6	7	19
Chicken Sliced	2 slices (57 g)	130	3	9	9
CHICKPEAS					
chickpeas	1 cup	285	54	3	12
Eden					
Organic	½ cup (4.1 oz)	110	17	2	6
Goya					
Spanish Style	7.5 oz	150	32	2	9
CHILI					
con carne w/ beans	8.9 oz	254	22	8	25
Allen					
Mexican Chili Beans	½ cup (4.5 oz)	120	22	1	6
Armour					
Chili No Beans	1 cup (8.7 oz)	470	18	38	14
Health Valley					
Mild Vegetarian With Lentils	5 oz	140	15	4	8
Hormel					
Chili Mac	1 can (7.5 oz)	200	17	9	11
Turkey Chili No Beans	1 cup (8.3 oz)	190	17	3	23
Micro Cup Meals					
Chili With Beans	1 cup (7.5 oz)	250	23	11	15
Van Camp's					
Chilee Beanee Weenee	1 can (8 oz)	240	27	12	14
CHIPS					
corn barbecue	1 oz	148	16	9	2
corn plain	1 oz	153	16	10	2
corn puffs cheese	1 oz	157	15	10	2
potato	1 oz	152	15	10	2
potato barbecue	1 oz	139	15	9	2
potato cheese	1 oz	140	16	8	2
potato light	1 oz	134	19	6	2
potato sour cream & onion	1 oz	150	15	10	2
potato sticks	½ cup (0.6 oz)	94	10	6	1

FOOD	PORTION	CALS.	CARB.	FAT	PRO.
taro	1 oz	141	19	7	1
tortilla nacho	1 oz	141	18	7	2
tortilla nacho light	1 bag (6 oz)	757	122	26	15
tortilla plain	1 oz	142	18	7	2
tortilla taco	1 oz	136	18	7	2
Eagle					
Potato Ridged	1 oz	150	15	10	2
Eden					
Vegetable Chips	50 (1 oz)	130	24	4	tr
Guiltless Gourmet					
Tortilla Baked	22-26 chips (1 oz)	110	21	1	3
Hain					
Carrot Chips	1 oz	150	16	9	2
Pringles					
Potato Original	14 chips (1 oz)	160	—	11	2
Potato Right Original	16 chips (1 oz)	140	—	7	1
Sunchips					
Multigrain	12 pieces (1 oz)	150	18	8	2
Terra Chips					
Sweet Potato	1 oz	140	18	7	1
Top Banana					
Plantain Chips	1 oz	150	17	8	1
Weight Watchers					
Potato Great Snackers Cheddar Cheese	½ oz	70	10	3	1

CHIVES

FOOD	PORTION	CALS.	CARB.	FAT	PRO.
fresh chopped	1 tbsp	1	tr	tr	tr

CHOCOLATE

FOOD	PORTION	CALS.	CARB.	FAT	PRO.
chips milk chocolate	1 cup (6 oz)	862	100	52	12
chips semisweet	1 cup (6 oz)	804	106	50	7
syrup chocolate	2 tbsp	82	22	tr	1
Quik					
Syrup Chocolate	1 ⅔ tbsp	100	22	1	1

CHUTNEY

FOOD	PORTION	CALS.	CARB.	FAT	PRO.
apple	1.2 oz	68	18	0	tr
tomato	1.2 oz	54	14	0	tr

CILANTRO

FOOD	PORTION	CALS.	CARB.	FAT	PRO.
fresh	¼ cup	1	tr	tr	tr

FOOD	PORTION	CALS.	CARB.	FAT	PRO.
CLAM JUICE					
Doxsee					
Clam Juice	3 fl oz	4	0	0	tr
CLAMS					
breaded & fried	¾ cup	451	39	26	13
cooked	20 sm	133	5	2	23
raw	9 lg (180 g)	133	5	2	23
raw	20 sm (180 g)	133	5	2	23
Doxsee					
Chopped Canned	6.5 oz	90	6	tr	16
COCOA					
hot cocoa	1 cup	218	26	9	9
COCONUT					
cream canned	1 tbsp	36	2	3	1
dried toasted	1 oz	168	13	13	2
fresh	1 piece (1½ oz)	159	7	15	2
COD					
atlantic cooked	3 oz	89	0	1	19
pacific baked	3 oz	95	0	1	21
COFFEE					
cafe au lait	1 cup (8 fl oz)	77	6	4	4
cafe brulot	1 cup (4.8 fl oz)	48	3	0	tr
cappuccino mix as prep	7 oz	62	11	2	tr
cappuccino	1 cup (8 fl oz)	77	6	4	4
coffee con leche	1 cup (8 fl oz)	77	6	4	4
espresso	1 cup (3 fl oz)	2	tr	0	tr
instant decaffeinated as prep	6 oz	4	1	0	tr
instant regular as prep	6 oz	4	1	0	tr
irish coffee	1 serv (9 fl oz)	107	3	3	1
mocha	1 mug (9.6 fl oz)	202	17	15	3
COFFEE SUBSTITUTES					
Postum					
Instant	6 oz	11	3	0	0
COFFEE WHITENERS					
Coffee-Mate					
Liquid	1 tbsp (0.5 fl oz)	16	2	1	0

FOOD	PORTION	CALS.	CARB.	FAT	PRO.
Weight Watchers					
Dairy Creamer Instant Nonfat Dry Milk	1 pkg	10	1	0	1

COLLARDS

cooked	½ cup	17	4	tr	1

COOKIES

FOOD	PORTION	CALS.	CARB.	FAT	PRO.
animal crackers	1 (2.5 g)	11	2	tr	tr
biscotti with nuts chocolate dipped	1 (1.3 oz)	117	16	6	2
butter	1 (5 g)	23	3	1	tr
chocolate chip	1 (0.4 oz)	48	7	2	1
chocolate chip low fat	1 (0.25 oz)	45	7	2	1
chocolate chip soft-type	1 (0.5 oz)	69	9	4	1
chocolate w/ creme filling	1 (0.35 oz)	47	7	2	1
chocolate w/ creme filling chocolate coated	1 (0.60 oz)	82	11	5	1
chocolate wafer	1 (0.2 oz)	26	4	1	tr
fig bars	1 (0.56 oz)	56	11	1	1
fortune	1 (0.28 oz)	30	7	tr	tr
fudge	1 (0.73 oz)	73	17	1	1
gingersnaps	1 (0.24 oz)	29	5	1	tr
graham	1 squares (0.24 oz)	30	5	1	1
graham chocolate covered	1 (0.49 oz)	68	9	3	1
marshmallow chocolate coated	1 (0.46 oz)	55	9	2	1
molasses	1 (0.5 oz)	65	11	2	1
oatmeal	1 (0.6 oz)	81	12	3	1
peanut butter sandwich	1 (0.5 oz)	67	9	3	1
shortbread	1 (0.28 oz)	40	5	2	1
sugar	1 (0.52 oz)	72	10	3	1
sugar wafers w/ creme filling	1 (0.12 oz)	18	3	1	tr
vanilla sandwich	1 (0.35 oz)	48	7	2	tr
Oreo					
Cookies	3 (1.2 oz)	160	23	7	2
Reduced Fat	3 (1.2 oz)	140	24	5	2
Snackwell's					
Fat Free Devil's Food	1 (0.5 oz)	50	13	0	1
Reduced Fat Chocolate Chip	13 (1 oz)	130	22	4	2

FOOD	PORTION	CALS.	CARB.	FAT	PRO.
Stella D'Oro					
Kichel Low Sodium	21	150	13	9	4
CORN					
cream style	½ cup	93	23	1	2
on-the-cob w/ butter cooked	1 ear	155	32	3	4
w/ red & green peppers canned	½ cup	86	21	1	3
yellow canned	½ cup	66	15	1	2
Ka-Me					
Baby	½ cup (4.5 oz)	20	3	0	1
Mrs. Paul's					
Fritters	2	240	35	9	5
Ore Ida					
Cob Corn	1 ear (6.1 oz)	180	33	3	6
Stouffer's					
Souffle	½ cup (2.4 oz)	170	21	7	5
CORNMEAL					
hush puppies	1 (¾ oz)	74	10	3	3
Aurora					
Polenta	½ cup (5 oz)	110	24	0	2
COTTAGE CHEESE					
creamed	1 cup	217	6	9	26
dry curd	1 cup	123	3	1	25
lowfat 1%	1 cup	164	6	2	28
lowfat 2%	1 cup	203	8	4	31
Axelrod					
Nonfat	½ cup (4.4 oz)	90	7	0	15
Breakstone					
Dry Curd ½% Fat	¼ cup (1.9 oz)	45	3	0	8
Hood					
4% Fat Pineapple	½ cup (4 oz)	130	15	4	10
Lactaid					
1%	4 oz	72	3	1	12
Light N'Lively					
Free	½ cup (4.4 oz)	80	5	0	14
COUSCOUS					
cooked	½ cup	101	21	tr	3
CRAB					
alaska king cooked	3 oz	82	0	1	16

FOOD	PORTION	CALS.	CARB.	FAT	PRO.
baked	1 (3.8 oz)	160	4	2	29
blue cooked	3 oz	87	0	2	17
canned	3 oz	84	0	1	17
crab cakes	1 cake (2.1 oz)	93	tr	5	12
soft-shell fried	1 (4.4 oz)	334	31	18	11

CRACKERS

FOOD	PORTION	CALS.	CARB.	FAT	PRO.
melba toast plain	1 (5 g)	19	4	tr	1
oyster cracker	1 (1 g)	4	1	tr	tr
saltines	1 (3 g)	13	2	tr	tr
saltines fat free low sodium	3 (0.5 oz)	59	12	tr	2
wheat thins	1 (2 g)	9	1	tr	tr
Adrienne's					
Gourmet Flatbread Classic Island	2	20	3	tr	1
Cheez-It					
Crackers	27 (1 oz)	160	16	8	4
Eden					
Brown Rice	5 (1 oz)	120	22	2	3
Hain					
Sourdough	½ oz	65	9	3	2
Health Valley					
Seven Grain Vegetable Stoned Wheat	13	55	9	2	1
Hi Ho					
Crackers	9	160	18	9	2
J.J. Flats					
Breadflats Plain	1	53	10	1	1
Keebler					
Toasted Snack Bacon	2	30	4	2	tr
Krispy					
Unsalted Tops	5 (0.5 oz)	60	10	2	2
Lavash					
Bread Crisp Original	2 (0.5 oz)	60	11	1	2
Manischewitz					
Tam Tams	10	147	17	8	2
NABS					
Peanut Butter Toast Sandwich	6 (1.4 oz)	190	24	10	4
Nabisco					
Royal Lunch	1 (0.4 oz)	50	8	2	tr

FOOD	PORTION	CALS.	CARB.	FAT	PRO.
Oysterettes					
Crackers	19 (0.5 oz)	60	10	3	1
Pepperidge Farm					
Goldfish Original	1 oz	130	18	5	3
Snack Mix Classic	1 oz	140	14	8	4
Premium					
Saltine Original	5 (0.5 oz)	60	10	2	1
Ritz					
Crackers	5 (0.5 oz)	80	10	4	1
Snackwell's					
Cracked Pepper	7 (0.5 oz)	60	13	0	2
Fat Free Wheat	5 (0.5 oz)	60	12	0	2
Reduced Fat Cheese	38 (1 oz)	130	23	2	4
Reduced Fat Classic Golden	6 (0.5 oz)	60	11	1	1
Tree Of Life					
Bite Size Fat Free Soya Nut	12	60	12	0	2
Triscuit					
Crackers	7 (1.1 oz)	140	21	5	3
Uneeda Biscuit					
Unsalted Tops	2 (0.5 oz)	60	11	2	1
Venus					
Water Crackers Fat Free	5 (0.5 oz)	55	11	0	2
Wasa Crispbread					
Extra Crisp	1	25	5	0	1
Wheatworth					
Stone Ground	5 (0.5 oz)	80	10	4	2
Zwieback					
Crackers	1 (8 g)	35	5	1	1
CRANBERRIES					
cranberry sauce sweetened	½ cup	209	54	tr	tr
fresh chopped	1 cup	54	14	tr	tr
S&W					
Cranberry Sauce Whole Berry Old Fashioned	½ cup	90	22	0	0
CRANBERRY BEANS					
cranberry beans	1 cup	216	39	1	14
CRANBERRY JUICE					
cranberry juice cocktail	6 oz	108	27	tr	0
cranberry juice cocktail low calorie	6 oz	33	9	0	0

FOOD	PORTION	CALS.	CARB.	FAT	PRO.
CREAM					
half & half	1 tbsp	20	1	2	tr
heavy whipping	1 tbsp	52	tr	6	tr
light coffee	1 cup	496	9	46	6
whipped	1 cup	411	7	44	5
CREAM CHEESE					
regular	1 oz	99	1	10	2
Alpine Lace					
Fat Free Garlic & Herbs	2 tbsp (1 oz)	30	1	tr	5
Breakstone					
Temp-Tee Whipped	3 tbsp (1.2 oz)	110	1	10	3
Healthy Choice					
Strawberry	2 tbsp (1 oz)	30	5	0	4
Philadelphia					
Free	1 oz	25	2	0	4
Free Soft	2 tbsp (1.2 oz)	30	2	0	5
Weight Watchers					
Reduced Fat	2 tbsp	35	1	2	3
CREAM CHEESE SUBSTITUTES					
Tofutti					
Better Than Cream Cheese French Onion	1 oz	80	1	8	1
CROISSANT					
cheese	1 (2 oz)	236	27	12	5
plain	1 (2 oz)	232	26	12	5
w/ egg & cheese	1	369	24	25	13
w/ egg cheese & bacon	1	413	24	28	16
w/ egg cheese & ham	1	475	24	34	19
w/ egg cheese & sausage	1	524	25	38	20
CROUTONS					
plain	1 cup (1 oz)	122	22	2	4
CUCUMBER					
cucumber salad	3.5 oz	50	11	tr	1
raw sliced	½ cup (1.8 oz)	7	1	tr	tr
CURRANTS					
zante dried	½ cup	204	53	tr	3

FOOD	PORTION	CALS.	CARB.	FAT	PRO.
CUSTARD					
baked	½ cup (5 oz)	148	15	7	7
flan	½ cup (5.4 oz)	220	35	6	7
zabaione	½ cup (57.2 g)	135	13	5	3
DANDELION GREENS					
fresh cooked	½ cup	17	3	tr	1
DANISH PASTRY					
almond	1, 4¼ in (2.3 oz)	280	30	16	5
cheese	1 (3 oz)	353	29	25	6
cinnamon nut	1, 4¼ in (2.3 oz)	280	30	16	5
fruit	1 (3.3 oz)	335	45	16	5
DATES					
whole	10	228	61	tr	2
DELI MEATS/COLD CUTS					
bologna beef	1 oz	88	tr	8	4
bologna beef & pork	1 oz	89	1	8	3
bologna pork	1 oz	70	tr	6	4
braunschweiger pork	1 oz	102	1	9	4
headcheese pork	1 oz	60	tr	5	5
liverwurst pork	1 oz	92	1	8	4
mortadella beef & pork	1 oz	88	1	7	5
olive loaf pork	1 oz	67	3	5	3
pepperoni pork & beef	1 slice (0.2 oz)	27	tr	2	1
salami cooked beef & pork	1 oz	71	1	6	4
salami hard pork	1 pkg (4 oz)	460	2	38	26
submarine w/ salami ham, cheese lettuce tomato onion & oil	1	456	51	19	22
Carl Buddig					
Corned Beef	1 oz	40	1	2	5
Pastrami	1 oz	40	1	2	5
DiLusso					
Genoa	1 oz	100	0	8	6
Healthy Choice					
Deli-Thin Bologna	4 slices (1.8 oz)	60	3	2	8
Hebrew National					
Bologna Beef Reduced Fat	2 oz	130	—	12	6
Salami Midget	2 oz	170	—	14	8

FOOD	PORTION	CALS.	CARB.	FAT	PRO.
Hillshire					
Flavor Pack 90-99% Fat Free Pastrami	1 slice (0.6 oz)	18	tr	tr	4
Lunch 'N Munch Pepperoni/ American	1 pkg (4.5 oz)	570	20	46	22
Jones					
Liver Sausage Chub	1 slice	80	tr	7	5
Oscar Mayer					
Bologna Light	1 slice (1 oz)	60	2	4	3
Lunchables Deluxe Turkey/Ham	1 pkg (5.1 oz)	360	23	19	23
Peppered Loaf	1 slice (1 oz)	39	1	2	5
Pickle And Pimiento Loaf	1 slice (1 oz)	70	2	6	3
Russer					
Jalapeno Loaf With Monterey Jack Cheese	2 oz	160	4	13	6
Polish Loaf	2 oz	140	7	10	7
Spam					
Original	2 oz	170	0	16	7

DINNER

FOOD	PORTION	CALS.	CARB.	FAT	PRO.
Armour					
Classics Chicken Parmigiana	1 meal (10.75 oz)	360	25	18	24
Classics Salisbury Steak	1 meal (11.25 oz)	330	20	18	23
Classics Swedish Meatballs	1 meal (10 oz)	300	20	17	18
Banquet					
Extra Helping All White Chicken	1 meal (18 oz)	820	72	41	40
Family Entree Beef Stew	1 serv (8.13 oz)	160	17	4	14
Hot Sandwich Toppers Creamed Chipped Beef	1 pkg (4 oz)	100	8	3	9
Budget Gourmet					
Beef Cantonese	1 meal (9.1 oz)	270	31	9	15
Chicken Marsala	1 meal (9 oz)	260	31	8	17
Teriyaki Beef	1 pkg (10.75 oz)	260	37	7	19
Healthy Choice					
Classics Mesquite Beef Barbecue	1 meal (11 oz)	310	45	4	23
Country Roast Turkey With Mushroom	1 meal (8.5 oz)	220	28	4	19
Traditional Beef Tips	1 meal (11.25 oz)	260	32	5	20

FOOD	PORTION	CALS.	CARB.	FAT	PRO.
Kid Cuisine					
Macaroni & Beef	1 pkg (9.6 oz)	370	58	9	12
Le Menu					
LightStyle Sweet & Sour Chicken	10 oz	250	29	7	18
Lean Cuisine					
Beef Pot Roast	1 meal (9 oz)	210	21	7	16
Meatloaf	1 pkg (9.4 oz)	270	24	10	21
Stuffed Cabbage	1 meal (9.5 oz)	220	27	7	11
Swedish Meatballs	1 pkg (9.1 oz)	290	32	8	22
Life Choice					
Garden Potato Casserole	1 meal (13.4 oz)	160	37	1	8
Morton					
Chicken Nugget	1 meal (7 oz)	320	30	17	13
Salisbury Steak	1 meal (9 oz)	210	23	9	9
Turkey	1 meal (9 oz)	230	27	8	14
My Own Meal					
Beef Stew	1 pkg (10 oz)	260	22	11	19
Stouffer's					
Chicken A La King	1 pkg (9.5 oz)	320	43	10	15
Homestyle Fish Filet With Macaroni & Cheese	1 pkg (9 oz)	430	37	21	24
Homestyle Veal Parmigiana	1 pkg (11.9 oz)	420	43	19	20
Lunch Express Stir-Fry Rice & Chicken	1 pkg (9 oz)	280	39	9	11
Swanson					
Chopped Sirloin Beef	10.75 oz	340	28	16	20
Fish 'n' Chips	10 oz	500	60	21	20
Homestyle Scalloped Potatoes & Ham	9 oz	300	26	13	19
Tyson					
Francais	1 pkg (9.5 oz)	280	20	14	19
Glazed Chicken With Sauce	1 pkg (9.25 oz)	240	29	4	22
Grilled Chicken	1 pkg (7.75 oz)	220	22	3	26
Ultra Slim-Fast					
Chicken Fettuccini	12 oz	380	38	12	31
Shrimp Creole	12 oz	240	45	4	12
Turkey Medallions In Herb Sauce	12 oz	280	33	6	23
Weight Watchers					
Beef Stroganoff	8.5 oz	280	29	9	21

FOOD	PORTION	CALS.	CARB.	FAT	PRO.
Weight Watchers (CONT.)					
Chicken Cordon Bleu	7.7 oz	170	15	5	19
Oven Baked Fish	7 oz	150	6	4	20

DIP

FOOD	PORTION	CALS.	CARB.	FAT	PRO.
Breakstone					
Sour Cream Chesapeake Clam	2 tbsp (1.1 oz)	50	2	4	1
Chi-Chi's					
Fiesta Bean	2 tbsp (0.9 oz)	35	4	2	1
Frito Lay					
French Onion	1 oz	50	3	4	1
Guiltless Gourmet					
Black Bean Spicy	1 oz	25	5	0	2
Hain					
Taco Dip & Sauce	4 tbsp	25	1	1	5
Heluva Good Cheese					
Ranch	2 tbsp (1.1 oz)	60	2	5	1
Knudsen					
Sour Cream Bacon & Onion	2 tbsp (1.1 oz)	60	2	5	1
Kraft					
Avocado	2 tbsp (1.1 oz)	60	4	4	1
Premium Creamy Cucumber	2 tbsp (1.1 oz)	50	2	4	tr
Louise's					
Fat Free Honey Mustard	1 oz	40	9	0	1
Marzetti					
Blue Cheese Veggie	2 tbsp	200	1	21	1
Old El Paso					
Chunky Salsa Medium	2 tbsp	10	1	0	1
Snyder's					
Mustard Pretzel	2 tbsp (1.2 oz)	90	13	4	1

DOUGHNUTS

FOOD	PORTION	CALS.	CARB.	FAT	PRO.
cake type unsugared	1 (1.6 oz)	198	23	11	2
chocolate glazed	1 (1.5 oz)	175	24	8	2
chocolate sugared	1 (1.5 oz)	175	24	8	2
chocolate coated	1 (1.5 oz)	204	21	13	2
creme filled	1 (3 oz)	307	26	21	6
french cruller glazed	1 (1.4 oz)	169	24	8	1
honey bun	1 (2.1 oz)	242	27	14	4
jelly	1 (3 oz)	289	33	16	5

FOOD	PORTION	CALS.	CARB.	FAT	PRO.
old fashioned	1 (1.6 oz)	198	23	11	2
wheat glazed	1 (1.6 oz)	162	19	9	3
yeast glazed	1 (2.1 oz)	242	27	14	4
Dutch Mill					
Cider	1 (2.1 oz)	240	35	10	3
Entenmann's					
Crumb Topped	1 (2.1 oz)	260	34	12	3
Hostess					
Gem Donettes Cinnamon	6 (3 oz)	320	53	11	5
O's Raspberry Filled Powdered	1 (2.2 oz)	230	35	10	3
Little Debbie					
Donut Sticks	1 pkg (3 oz)	390	45	23	4
Tastykake					
Cinnamon	1 (47 g)	180	26	8	3
DRINK MIXERS					
whiskey sour mix as prep	3.6 oz	169	16	0	tr
Bacardi					
Margarita Mix w/o liquor	8 fl oz	100	25	0	0
Pina Colada	8 fl oz	140	34	0	0
Strawberry Daiquiri w/o liquor	8 fl oz	140	35	0	0
Canada Dry					
Sour Mixer	8 fl oz	90	22	0	0
Libby					
Bloody Mary Mix	6 oz	40	8	0	2
DUCK					
w/ skin roasted	½ duck (13.4 oz)	1287	0	108	73
w/o skin roasted	½ duck (7.8 oz)	445	0	25	52
EEL					
smoked	3.5 oz	330	0	28	19
EGG					
fried w/ margarine	1	91	1	7	6
hard cooked	1	77	1	5	6
poached	1	74	1	5	6
scrambled w/ whole milk & margarine	1	101	1	7	7
EGG DISHES					
deviled	2 halves	145	1	13	6
salad	½ cup	307	2	28	13

FOOD	PORTION	CALS.	CARB.	FAT	PRO.
sandwich w/ cheese	1	340	26	19	16
sandwich w/ cheese & ham	1	348	31	16	19
EGG SUBSTITUTES					
Egg Beaters					
Eggs Substitute	¼ cup	25	1	0	5
Morningstar Farms					
Scramblers	¼ cup (57 g)	60	3	3	6
EGGNOG					
eggnog	1 cup	342	34	19	10
Borden					
Light	½ cup	130	23	2	5
Hood					
Fat Free	4 fl oz	100	21	0	4
EGGPLANT					
baba ghannouj	¼ cup	55	5	4	2
slices cooked	4 (7 oz)	38	0	0	2
Mrs. Paul's					
Parmigiana	5 oz	240	18	16	6
Progresso					
Caponata	2 tbsp (1 oz)	30	2	2	0
ENDIVE					
raw chopped	½ cup	4	1	tr	tr
ENGLISH MUFFIN					
plain	1	134	26	1	4
w/ butter	1	189	30	6	5
w/ cheese & sausage	1	394	29	24	15
w/ egg cheese & bacon	1	487	31	31	22
w/ egg cheese & canadian bacon	1	383	31	20	20
FALAFEL					
falafel	1 (1.2 oz)	57	5	3	2
FAVA BEANS					
Progresso					
Canned	½ cup	90	15	tr	7
FENNEL					
fresh sliced	1 cup	27	6	tr	1
FIGS					
dried whole	10	477	122	2	6
fresh	1 med	50	10	tr	tr

FOOD	PORTION	CALS.	CARB.	FAT	PRO.
FISH					
fish cake	1 (4.7 oz)	166	6	7	18
sandwich w/ tartar sauce	1	431	41	55	17
sandwich w/ tartar sauce & cheese	1	524	48	29	21
taramasalata	3.5 oz	446	4	46	3
Holmes					
Finest Kippered Snacks drained	1 can (3.2 oz)	135	0	8	17
Port Clyde					
Fish Steaks In Mustard Sauce	1 can (3.75 oz)	140	1	7	18
FISH SUBSTITUTES					
Worthington					
Fillets	2 (85 g)	180	9	9	15
FLOUNDER					
battered & fried	3.2 oz	211	15	11	13
breaded & fried	3.2 oz	211	15	11	13
cooked	3 oz	99	0	1	21
FRENCH TOAST					
w/ butter	2 slices	356	36	19	10
FROG'S LEGS					
frog leg as prep w/ seasoned flour & fried	1 (0.8)	70	15	5	4
FRUIT DRINKS					
After The Fall					
Mango Montage	1 bottle (10 oz)	140	33	0	1
Strawberry Vanilla	1 can (12 oz)	160	42	0	tr
Boku					
White Grape Raspberry	16 fl oz	120	29	0	0
Bright & Early					
Fruit Punch	8 fl oz	130	31	0	0
Crystal Geyser					
Juice Squeeze Wild Berry	1 bottle (12 fl oz)	130	31	0	1
Crystal Light					
Lemon-Lime	8 oz	4	0	0	0
Dole					
Pineapple Grapefruit as prep	8 fl oz	130	29	0	1
Pineapple Orange	6 fl oz	90	22	0	0
Five Alive					
Citrus Chilled	8 fl oz	120	30	0	0

FOOD	PORTION	CALS.	CARB.	FAT	PRO.
Five Alive (CONT.)					
Tropical Citrus	8 fl oz	120	29	0	0
Hi-C					
Boppin' Berry	8 fl oz	130	32	0	0
Hula Punch	8 fl oz	120	29	0	0
Hood					
Natural Blenders Apple Peach Pear	1 cup (8 oz)	120	30	0	0
Juicy Juice					
Tropical	1 bottle (6 fl oz)	110	26	0	1
Kern's					
Apricot Pineapple Nectar	6 fl oz	110	27	0	0
Kool-Aid					
Koolers Sharkleberry Fin	1 pkg (8.45 fl oz)	140	37	0	0
Sugar Free Rainbow Punch	8 oz	4	0	0	0
Sugar Sweetened Rainbow Punch	8 oz	84	21	0	0
Lifesavers					
Lime Punch	8 fl oz	140	34	0	0
Mauna La'i					
Mango & Hawaiian Guava Fruit Juice Drink	8 fl oz	130	33	0	0
Minute Maid					
Berry Punch Box	8.45 fl oz	130	31	0	0
Juices To Go Concord Punch	1 can (11.5 fl oz)	180	46	0	0
Tropical Punch	8 fl oz	120	31	0	0
Mott's					
Apple Cranberry Blend	10 fl oz	180	44	0	0
Ocean Spray					
Cran.Blueberry	8 fl oz	160	41	0	0
Odwalla					
Mango Tango	8 fl oz	150	37	3	1
Mo Beta	16 fl oz	280	69	1	3
Pek					
Mango Guava Ecstasy	1 bottle (20 fl oz)	110	27	0	0
S&W					
Apricot Pineapple Nectar	6 fl oz	120	29	0	1
Apricot Pineapple Nectar Diet	6 fl oz	80	20	0	0
Seneca					
Raspberry-Cranberry Juice Cocktail frzn as prep	8 fl oz	140	36	0	0

FOOD	PORTION	CALS.	CARB.	FAT	PRO.
Smucker's					
Orange Banana	8 oz	120	30	0	0
Snapple					
Diet Kiwi Strawberry	8 fl oz	13	3	0	0
Squeezit					
Mean Green Puncher	1 (6.75 fl oz)	90	23	0	0
Tree Top					
Apple Pear as prep	6 oz	90	22	0	0
Apple Raspberry	6 fl oz	80	21	0	0
Tropicana					
Citrus Punch	8 fl oz	140	36	0	0
Pineapple Punch	8 fl oz	120	31	0	0
Season's Best Cranberry Medley	8 fl oz	120	29	0	tr
Tropics Orange Kiwi Passion	8 fl oz	100	26	0	tr
Veryfine					
Papaya Punch	8 fl oz	120	30	0	0
Wylers					
Drink Mix Unsweetened Pink	8 fl oz	3	1	0	0
FRUIT MIXED					
fruit cocktail juice pack	½ cup	56	15	tr	1
fruit cocktail water pack	½ cup	40	10	tr	1
fruit salad in light syrup	½ cup	73	19	tr	tr
fruit salad juice pack	½ cup	62	16	tr	1
Big Valley					
Cup A Fruit	1 pkg (4 oz)	50	7	0	tr
Del Monte					
Dried Mixed	⅓ cup (1.4 oz)	110	30	0	0
Snack Cups Mixed Fruit Fruit Naturals	1 serv (4.5 oz)	60	16	0	0
Sonoma					
Trail Mix	¼ cup (1.4 oz)	160	24	7	3
FRUIT SNACKS					
fruit leather	1 bar (0.8 oz)	81	18	1	tr
fruit leather rolls	1 lg (0.7 oz)	73	18	1	tr
Betty Crocker					
String Thing Cherry	1 pkg (0.7 oz)	80	17	1	0
Del Monte					
Sierra Trail Mix	¼ cup (1.2 oz)	150	20	8	4

FOOD	PORTION	CALS.	CARB.	FAT	PRO.
Fruit Roll-Ups					
Strawberry	1 (½ oz)	50	12	tr	tr
Health Valley					
Bakes Apple	1 bar	100	16	3	2
Fat Free Fruit Bars 100% Organic Raisin	1 bar	140	33	tr	3
Fruit & Fitness Bars	2 bars	200	35	5	4
Oat Bran Bakes Fig & Nut	1 bar	110	16	3	2
Rice Bran Jumbo Fruit Bars Almond & Date	1 bar	160	27	5	3
Sovex					
Fruit Bites Jungle Pals	1 pkg (0.9 oz)	90	21	1	0
Stretch Island					
Fruit Leather Organic Grape	2 pieces (1 oz)	90	24	0	0
Sunbelt					
Fruit Boosters Blueberry	1 (1.3 oz)	130	27	2	1
Sunkist					
Fruit Roll Cherry	1	75	18	tr	tr
Weight Watchers					
Peach	½ oz	50	13	tr	tr
GARLIC					
clove	1	4	1	tr	tr
GEFILTE FISH					
sweet	1 piece (1.5 oz)	35	3	1	4
GELATIN					
low calorie	½ cup	8	0	0	2
mix as prep	½ cup (4.7 oz)	80	19	0	2
Del Monte					
Gel Snack Cups Orange	1 serv (3.5 oz)	70	19	0	0
Gel Snack Cups Strawberry	1 serv (3.5 oz)	70	19	0	0
Knox					
Orange Flavored Drinking Gelatin w/ Nutrasweet	1 pkg	39	4	tr	6
Kojel					
Diet	1 serv	10	4	tr	1
GOAT					
roasted	3 oz	122	0	3	23

FOOD	PORTION	CALS.	CARB.	FAT	PRO.
GOOSE					
w/ skin roasted	6.6 oz	574	0	41	47
w/o skin roasted	5 oz	340	0	18	41
GRANOLA BARS					
Carnation					
Honey & Oats	1 (1.26 oz)	130	23	4	2
Fi-Bar					
Peanut Butter	1	130	20	4	3
General Mills					
Nature Valley Oats N'Honey	1	120	17	5	2
Grist Mill					
Chew Chocolate Chip	1 (1 oz)	130	21	4	2
Hershey					
Chocolate Covered Chocolate Chip	1 (1.2 oz)	170	22	8	2
Kellogg's					
Low Fat Crunchy Cinnamon Raisin	1 (0.7 oz)	80	16	2	2
Kudos					
Chocolate Coated Milk & Cookies	1 (1 oz)	130	18	5	2
New Country					
Chocolate Covered Cookies & Creme	1	200	23	11	2
Quaker					
Dipps Caramel Nut	1	148	21	6	2
Sunbelt					
Chewy With Almonds	1 (1.5 oz)	190	25	10	3
GRANOLA CEREAL					
Erewhon					
Maple	1 oz	130	17	5	3
General Mills					
Nature Valley Fruit & Nut	⅓ cup (1 oz)	130	19	5	2
Good Shepherd					
Organic 5 Grain Muesli	1 oz	160	27	3	4
Organic Wheat Free Blueberry Amaranth	1 oz	110	22	1	3
Grist Mill					
Low-Fat With Raisins	⅔ cup (1.9 oz)	220	42	3	5
Kellogg's					
Low Fat	½ cup (1.9 oz)	210	43	3	5

FOOD	PORTION	CALS.	CARB.	FAT	PRO.
Sunbelt					
Banana Nut	1.9 oz	250	37	9	5
Uncle Roy's					
Cashew Raisin	½ cup (1.6 oz)	180	32	6	8
Organic Golden Honey	½ cup (1.6 oz)	190	30	6	5
GRAPE JUICE					
bottled	1 cup	155	38	tr	1
grape drink	6 oz	84	22	0	0
Kool-Aid					
Sugar Free	8 oz	3	0	0	0
Minute Maid					
Punch Chilled	8 fl oz	130	32	0	0
Seneca					
White Grape Juice frzn as prep	8 fl oz	140	33	0	0
GRAPE LEAVES					
Cedar's					
Grape Leaves Stuffed With Rice	6 pieces (4.9 oz)	180	22	8	4
GRAPEFRUIT					
juice pack jarred	½ cup	46	11	tr	1
pink	½	37	9	tr	1
red	½	37	9	tr	1
white	½	39	10	tr	1
GRAPEFRUIT JUICE					
fresh	1 cup	96	23	tr	1
frzn as prep	1 cup	102	24	tr	1
Minute Maid					
Juices To Go Pink Cocktail	1 bottle (16 fl oz)	110	27	0	0
GRAPES					
fresh	10	36	9	tr	tr
GRAVY					
Franco-American					
Au Jus	2 oz	10	2	0	0
Beef	2 oz	25	4	1	0
Chicken	2 oz	45	3	4	0
Mushroom	2 oz	25	3	1	0
Pork	2 oz	40	3	3	0
Turkey	2 oz	30	3	2	0

FOOD	PORTION	CALS.	CARB.	FAT	PRO.
GREAT NORTHERN BEANS					
cooked	1 cup	210	37	1	15
GREEN BEANS					
Birds Eye					
In Sauce French Green Beans With Toasted Almonds	½ cup	50	8	2	3
Del Monte					
Cut	½ cup (4.3 oz)	20	4	0	1
S&W					
Dilled	½ cup	60	15	0	1
Stouffer's					
Green Bean Mushroom Casserole	½ cup (1.9 oz)	130	13	8	3
GROUPER					
cooked	3 oz	100	0	1	21
GUANABANA JUICE					
Libby					
Nectar	1 can (11.5 fl oz)	210	50	0	0
GUAVA					
fresh	1	45	11	1	1
guava sauce	½ cup	43	11	tr	tr
GUAVA JUICE					
Kern's					
Nectar	6 fl oz	110	28	0	0
HADDOCK					
cooked	3 oz	95	0	1	21
smoked	3 oz	99	0	1	21
HALIBUT					
atlantic & pacific cooked	3 oz	119	0	2	23
greenland baked	3 oz	203	0	15	16
HAM					
Alpine Lace					
Boneless Cooked	2 oz	60	1	2	9
Armour					
Deviled Ham canned	1 pkg (3 oz)	200	0	16	14
Carl Buddig					
Honey Ham	1 oz	50	1	3	5

FOOD	PORTION	CALS.	CARB.	FAT	PRO.
Hansel n'Gretel					
Baked Virginia	1 oz	34	2	1	5
Healthy Choice					
Deli-Thin Cooked	6 slices (2 oz)	60	1	2	10
Hillshire					
Brown Sugar	1 oz	40	2	2	4
Deli Select Lower Salt	1 slice	10	tr	tr	2
Hormel					
Curemaster	3 oz	80	0	3	14
Ham & Cheese Patties	1 patty (2 oz)	190	0	17	7
Krakus					
Ham	1 oz	25	1	1	5
Louis Rich					
Dinner Slices Baked	1 slice (3.3 oz)	80	1	2	16
Oscar Mayer					
Chopped	1 slice (1 oz)	50	1	4	4
Deli-Thin Smoked	4 slices (1.8 oz)	50	0	2	9
Lower Sodium	3 slices (2.2 oz)	70	2	3	10
Lunchables Cookies/Ham/ Swiss	1 pkg (4.2 oz)	360	29	19	18
Lunchables Ham/Garden Vegetable Cheese	1 pkg (4.5 oz)	380	36	21	13
Russer					
Canadian Brand Maple	2 oz	70	4	2	9
Sara Lee					
Bavarian Brand Baked Honey	2 oz	80	2	4	9
Underwood					
Deviled	2.08 oz	220	tr	19	8
Deviled Light	2.08 oz	120	1	8	11
Weight Watchers					
Deli Thin Oven Roasted	5 slices (⅓ oz)	12	tr	tr	2
HAM DISHES					
croquettes	1 (3.1 oz)	217	11	14	12
salad	½ cup	287	5	23	16
sandwich w/ cheese	1	353	33	15	21
Hot Pocket					
Stuffed Sandwich Ham & Cheese	1 (4.5 ox)	340	37	15	14
HAMBURGER					
double patty w/ bun	1 reg	544	43	28	30

FOOD	PORTION	CALS.	CARB.	FAT	PRO.
double patty w/ catsup mayonnaise onion pickle tomato & bun	1 reg	649	53	35	30
double patty w/ catsup cheese mayonnaise mustard pickle tomato & bun	1 lg	706	40	44	38
double patty w/ cheese & bun	1 reg	457	22	28	28
double patty w/ cheese & double bun	1 reg	461	44	22	22
single patty w/ bacon catsup cheese mustard onion pickle & bun	1 lg	609	37	37	32
single patty w/ bun	1 lg	400	25	23	23
single patty w/ bun	1 reg	275	31	12	12
single patty w/ catsup cheese ham mayonnaise pickle tomato & bun	1 lg	745	38	48	40
single patty w/ cheese & bun	1 lg	608	47	33	30
triple patty w/ catsup mustard pickle & bun	1 lg	693	29	41	50
triple patty w/ cheese & bun	1 lg	769	27	51	56
HAZELNUTS					
oil roasted unblanched	1 oz	187	5	18	4
HEART					
chicken simmered	1 cup (5 oz)	268	tr	11	11
HEARTS OF PALM					
canned	1 (1.2 oz)	9	2	tr	1
HERRING					
atlantic kippered	1 fillet (1.4 oz)	87	0	5	10
atlantic cooked	3 oz	172	0	10	20
atlantic pickled	½ oz	39	1	3	2
HOMINY					
canned	½ cup	57	11	tr	1
HONEY					
honey	1 tbsp (0.7 oz)	64	17	0	tr
Tree Of Life					
Alfalfa	1 tbsp (0.7 oz)	60	17	0	0
Buckwheat	1 tbsp (0.7 oz)	60	17	0	0
Tupelo	1 tbsp (0.7 oz)	60	17	0	0
HONEYDEW					
cubed	1 cup	60	16	tr	1
wedge	⅒	46	12	tr	1

FOOD	PORTION	CALS.	CARB.	FAT	PRO.
HORSERADISH					
Gold's					
White	1 tsp	4	tr	tr	tr
Ka-Me					
Wasabi Powder	¼ tsp (1 g)	0	1	0	0
Kraft					
Cream Style	1 tsp (0.2 oz)	0	0	0	0
Rosoff's					
Red	1 tbsp (0.5 oz)	8	2	0	0
HOT DOG					
beef	1 (2 oz)	180	1	16	7
beef & pork	1 (2 oz)	183	1	17	6
chicken	1 (1.5 oz)	116	3	9	6
corndog	1	460	56	19	17
turkey	1 (1.5 oz)	102	1	8	6
w/ bun chili	1	297	31	13	14
w/ bun plain	1	242	18	15	10
Hebrew National					
Cocktail Beef	6 (1.8 oz)	160	—	15	6
Reduced Fat Beef	1 (1.7 oz)	120	—	10	5
Oscar Mayer					
Free	1 (1.8 oz)	40	2	0	7
Healthy Favorites Turkey & Beef	1 (2 oz)	60	2	2	9
Tyson					
Chicken Cheese	1	145	1	11	7
HUMMUS					
hummus	⅓ cup	140	17	7	4
ICE CREAM AND FROZEN DESSERTS					
cone vanilla light soft serve	1 (4.6 oz)	164	24	6	4
gelato chocolate hazelnut	½ cup (5.3 oz)	370	26	29	9
gelato vanilla	½ cup (3 oz)	211	18	15	3
3 Musketeers					
Single Vanilla	1 (2 fl oz)	160	16	10	2
Ben & Jerry's					
Cherry Garcia	½ cup (3.7 oz)	240	25	16	4
Bon Bons					
Vanilla With Milk Chocolate Coating	5 pieces	200	17	14	2

FOOD	PORTION	CALS.	CARB.	FAT	PRO.
Borden					
Buttered Pecan	½ cup	180	16	12	3
Fat Free Strawberry	½ cup	90	21	tr	2
Bounty					
Coconut/Dark	1 (0.84 fl oz)	70	7	5	1
Bresler's					
All Flavors Ice Cream	3.5 oz	230	23	12	3
Breyers					
Cherry Vanilla	½ cup	150	17	7	3
Reduced Fat Heavenly Hash	½ cup (2.4 oz)	150	22	5	4
Carnation					
Sundae Cup Strawberry	1 (3.3 oz)	200	29	8	2
DoveBar					
Crunchy Cookie	1 (3.8 fl oz)	340	35	21	4
Drumstick					
Cone Vanilla Fudge	1 (4.6 oz)	370	40	21	6
Edy's					
American Dream Vanilla	3 oz	80	18	tr	2
Light Vanilla	4 oz	100	13	4	3
Fi-Bar					
Banana Cream	1 bar	93	21	tr	2
Friendly's					
Fudge Nut Brownie	½ cup	200	23	11	3
Frusen Gladje					
Chocolate	½ cup	240	17	17	5
Good Humor					
Chocolate Eclair Classic	1 (3.1 fl oz)	170	21	9	2
King Cone Classic Vanilla	1 (4.8 oz)	300	48	10	4
Light Chocolate Chip	½ cup (2.4 oz)	130	20	4	3
Sandwich Ice Cream	1	190	28	8	3
Haagen-Dazs					
Chocolate Chocolate Chip	½ cup (3.7 oz)	300	26	20	5
Rum Raisin	½ cup (3.7 oz)	270	22	17	4
Healthy Choice					
Bordeaux Cherry Chocolate Chip	½ cup (2.5 oz)	110	19	2	3
Mint Chocolate Chip	½ cup (2.5 oz)	120	21	2	3
Hood					
Caramel Butterscotch Blast	½ cup (2.3 oz)	160	20	8	2

FOOD	PORTION	CALS.	CARB.	FAT	PRO.
Hood (CONT.)					
Fat Free Praline Pecan Delight	½ cup (2.5 oz)	120	27	0	2
Fat Free Vanilla Fudge Twist	½ cup (2.5 oz)	120	26	0	2
Klondike					
Original Bar	1 (5.2 fl oz)	290	24	20	3
Mocha Mix					
Neapolitan	½ cup (2.3 oz)	140	18	7	1
Rice Dream					
Cocoa Marble Fudge	½ cup	140	19	6	1
Sealtest					
Candy Cane Crunch	½ cup (2.4 oz)	150	21	6	2
Free Strawberry	½ cup	100	23	0	2
Maple Walnut	½ cup (2.4 oz)	160	16	9	3
Simple Pleasures					
Vanilla Fudge Swirl Light	4 oz	90	20	tr	5
Tofu Ice Creme					
Carob	4 fl oz	190	28	8	2
Turkey Hill					
Choco Mint Chip	½ cup (2.3 oz)	160	17	10	2
Ultra Slim-Fast					
Vanilla	4 oz	90	19	tr	5
Weight Watchers					
Bar Fat Free Vanilla Sandwich	1 (2.5 oz)	130	30	0	3
ICE CREAM TOPPINGS					
walnuts in syrup	2 tbsp (1.4 oz)	167	22	9	2
Hershey					
Chocolate Fudge	2 tbsp	100	14	4	1
ICE TEA					
Arizona					
Raspberry	8 fl oz	95	25	0	0
Royal Mistic					
Diet	12 fl oz	8	2	0	0
Snapple					
Lemon	8 fl oz	110	27	0	0
ICES AND ICE POPS					
fruit & juice bar	1 (3 fl oz)	75	19	tr	1
ice pop	1 (2 fl oz)	42	11	0	0

FOOD	PORTION	CALS.	CARB.	FAT	PRO.
JAM/JELLY/PRESERVES					
all flavors jam	1 tbsp (0.7 oz)	48	13	0	tr
all flavors jelly	1 tbsp (0.7 oz)	52	14	0	tr
all flavors preserve	1 tbsp (0.7 oz)	48	13	0	tr
apple butter	1 tbsp (0.6 oz)	33	9	0	0
KALE					
chopped cooked	½ cup	21	4	tr	1
KEFIR					
kefir	3½ oz	66	5	4	3
KIDNEY					
beef simmered	3 oz	122	0	3	22
KIDNEY BEANS					
cooked	1 cup	208	38	1	13
Eden					
Organic	½ cup (4.4 oz)	100	18	0	8
KIWIS					
fresh	1 med	46	11	tr	1
Sonoma					
Dried	7-8 pieces (1 oz)	90	19	1	2
KNISH					
kashe	1 (7 oz)	270	45	8	7
potato	1 lg (7 oz)	332	49	12	8
KOHLRABI					
raw sliced	½ cup	19	4	tr	1
sliced cooked	½ cup	24	5	tr	1
KUMQUATS					
fresh	1	12	3	tr	tr
LAMB					
cubed lean only braised	3 oz	190	0	7	29
cubed lean only broiled	3 oz	158	0	6	24
ground broiled	3 oz	240	0	17	21
loin chop w/ bone lean & fat Choice broiled	1 chop (2.3 oz)	201	0	15	16
rib chop lean & fat Choice broiled	3 oz	307	0	25	19
shank lean & fat Choice braised	3 oz	206	0	11	24
LAMB DISHES					
curry	¾ cup	345	22	17	26

FOOD	PORTION	CALS.	CARB.	FAT	PRO.
moussaka	5.6 oz	312	16	21	15
stew	¾ cup	124	11	5	10
LAMB'S-QUARTERS					
chopped cooked	½ cup	29	5	1	3
LEEKS					
cooked	1 (4.4 oz)	38	9	tr	1
LEMON					
wedge	1	5	3	tr	tr
LEMON CURD					
lemon curd made w/ egg	2 tsp	29	4	1	tr
LEMON JUICE					
fresh	1 tbsp	4	1	0	tr
LEMONADE					
Fruitopia					
Lemonade	8 fl oz	120	29	0	0
Minute Maid					
Juices To Go	1 bottle (16 fl oz)	110	28	0	0
Newman's Own					
Roadside Virginia	8 fl oz	100	22	tr	tr
Snapple					
Lemonade	8 fl oz	110	29	0	0
Tropicana					
Lemonade	1 can (11.5 oz)	160	39	0	tr
LENTILS					
cooked	1 cup	231	40	1	18
LETTUCE					
boston	2 leaves	2	tr	tr	tr
iceberg	1 leaf	3	tr	tr	tr
looseleaf shredded	½ cup	5	1	tr	tr
romaine shredded	½ cup	4	1	tr	tr
LIMA BEANS					
canned	½ cup	93	17	tr	6
LIME JUICE					
Realime					
Juice	1 oz	6	2	0	0
LIVER					
beef pan-fried	3 oz	184	7	7	23
chicken stewed	1 cup (5 oz)	219	1	8	34

FOOD	PORTION	CALS.	CARB.	FAT	PRO.
LOBSTER					
cooked	1 cup	142	2	1	30
newburg	1 cup	485	13	27	46
steamed	1 (5.7 oz)	233	5	3	43
LYCHEES					
fresh	1	6	2	tr	tr
Ka-Me					
Whole Pitted In Syrup	15 pieces (5 oz)	130	32	0	0
MACADAMIA NUTS					
oil roasted	1 oz	204	4	22	2
MACKEREL					
atlantic cooked	3 oz	223	0	15	20
canned	1 cup	296	0	12	44
MALT					
nonalcoholic	12 fl oz	32	5	0	1
MALTED MILK					
chocolate as prep w/ milk	1 cup	229	30	9	9
MANGO					
fresh	1	135	35	1	1
MANGO JUICE					
Libby					
Nectar	1 can (11.5 fl oz)	210	52	0	0
Snapple					
Mango Madness Cocktail	8 fl oz	110	29	0	0
MARGARINE					
stick corn	1 tsp	34	0	4	0
tub diet	1 tsp	17	0	2	0
MARSHMALLOW					
marshmallow	1 reg (0.3 oz)	23	6	0	tr
MATZO					
plain	1 (1 oz)	112	24	tr	3
whole wheat	1 (1 oz)	99	22	tr	4
MAYONNAISE					
mayonnaise	1 tbsp	99	tr	11	tr
Hellman's					
Chlesterol Free Reduced Calorie	1 tbsp (15 g)	50	1	5	0

FOOD	PORTION	CALS.	CARB.	FAT	PRO.
Kraft					
Free	1 tbsp (0.6 oz)	10	2	0	0
MAYONNAISE TYPE SALAD DRESSING					
Miracle Whip					
Free	1 tbsp (0.6 oz)	15	3	0	0
Salad Dressing	1 tbsp (0.5 oz)	70	2	7	0
MEAT STICKS					
jerky beef	1 oz	96	4	4	11
MEAT SUBSTITUTES					
Boca Burgers					
Original	1 patty (2.5 oz)	110	9	2	14
Green Giant					
Harvest Burgers Original	1 (3 oz)	140	8	4	18
Ken & Robert's					
Veggie Burger	1 (62 g)	110	19	2	5
Knox Mountain Farm					
Wheat Balls Mix	1 serv (1/10 pkg)	110	9	1	14
LaLoma					
Nuteena	½ in slice (65 g)	160	6	12	8
Sizzle Burger	1 patty (71 g)	220	10	12	17
Lightlife					
Smart Deli Slices	2 slices (1.5 oz)	44	1	0	8
Smart Dogs	1 (1.5 oz)	40	1	0	8
Morningstar Farms					
Sandwich Pattie Biscuit	1 (3.5 oz)	280	31	11	13
Natural Touch					
Garden Pattie	1 (67 g)	120	8	4	11
White Wave					
Meatless Jumbo Franks	1 (3 oz)	170	11	3	26
Veggie Burger	1 patty (2.5 oz)	110	16	3	5
Worthington					
Protose	½ in slice (76 g)	180	9	8	17
Vegetarian Burger	½ cup (113 g)	150	9	4	19
MILK					
1%	1 cup	102	12	3	8
1% protein fortified	1 cup	119	14	3	10
2%	1 cup	121	12	5	8
buttermilk	1 cup	99	12	2	8

FOOD	PORTION	CALS.	CARB.	FAT	PRO.
condensed sweetened	1 oz	123	21	3	3
goat	1 cup	168	11	10	9
skim	1 cup	86	12	tr	8
whole	1 cup	150	11	8	8
Borden					
Acidophilus 1%	8 fl oz	100	11	2	8
Hi-Protein 2%	8 fl oz	140	13	5	10
CalciMilk					
CalciMilk	8 fl oz	102	12	3	8
Carnation					
Evaporated	2 tbsp	40	3	3	2
Evaporated Lowfat	2 tbsp	25	3	1	2
Lite Evaporated Skimmed	½ cup (4 fl oz)	100	14	tr	9
Lactaid					
Nonfat	8 fl oz	86	12	tr	8
Parmalat					
1%	1 cup (8 oz)	110	13	3	9

MILK DRINKS

chocolate milk	1 cup	208	26	8	8

MILK SUBSTITUTES

Better Than Milk					
Carob	8 fl oz	130	20	5	2
Eden					
Original	1 pkg (8.8 oz)	135	14	4	10
EdenBlend					
Original	8 fl oz	120	16	3	7
EdenRice					
Drink	8 fl oz	110	21	3	1
Edensoy					
Vanilla	8 fl oz	150	23	3	6
Health Valley					
Soo Moo	1 cup	120	12	6	6
Rice Dream					
Lite Organic Original	8 fl oz	130	28	2	1
Spring Creek					
Original	1 oz	21	3	5	2
Vegelicious					
Drink	8 fl oz	100	18	2	2

FOOD	PORTION	CALS.	CARB.	FAT	PRO.
Vitasoy					
Original Creamy	8 fl oz	100	10	5	7
Original Light	8 fl oz	90	15	2	4
Westsoy					
Plain Lite	8 fl oz	100	16	2	4
MILKSHAKE					
chocolate	10 oz	360	58	11	10
strawberry	10 oz	319	53	8	10
vanilla	10 oz	314	51	8	10
MINERAL/BOTTLED WATER					
Evian					
Water	1 liter	0	0	0	0
MISO					
miso	½ cup	284	39	8	16
MOLASSES					
blackstrap	1 tbsp (0.7 oz)	47	12	0	0
molasses	1 tbsp (0.7 oz)	53	14	0	0
MONKFISH					
baked	3 oz	82	0	2	16
MOUSSE					
chocolate	½ cup (7.1 oz)	447	33	33	9
MUFFIN					
blueberry	1 (2 oz)	158	27	4	3
corn	1 (2 oz)	174	29	5	3
Dutch Mill					
Raisin Bran	1 (2 oz)	230	37	5	2
Weight Watchers					
Lemon Poppy Seed	1 (2.5 oz)	200	37	5	4
MUNG BEANS					
canned	½ cup	8	1	tr	1
stir fried	½ cup	31	7	tr	3
MUSHROOMS					
chanterelle	3½ oz	11	tr	tr	2
enoki raw	1 (4 in)	2	tr	tr	tr
morel	3½ oz	9	0	tr	2
oyster	3.5 oz	11	0	tr	2
pieces canned	½ cup	19	4	tr	1

FOOD	PORTION	CALS.	CARB.	FAT	PRO.
raw sliced	½ cup	9	2	tr	1
shitake cooked	4 (2.5 oz)	40	10	tr	1
Ka-Me					
Straw Whole Peeled	½ cup (4.5 oz)	20	3	0	2
MUSSELS					
blue raw	1 cup	129	6	3	18
fresh blue cooked	3 oz	147	6	4	20
MUSTARD					
yellow ready-to-use	1 tsp	5	tr	tr	tr
MUSTARD GREENS					
chopped cooked	½ cup	11	1	tr	2
NAVY BEANS					
cooked	1 cup	296	54	1	20
NECTARINE					
fresh	1	67	16	1	1
NEUFCHATEL					
neufchatel	1 oz	74	1	7	3
NOODLES					
cellophane	1 cup	492	121	tr	tr
chow mein	1 cup	237	26	14	4
egg cooked	1 cup	212	40	2	8
japanese soba cooked	½ cup	56	12	tr	3
japanese somen cooked	½ cup	115	24	tr	4
noodle pudding	½ cup	132	11	7	6
spinach/egg cooked	1 cup	211	39	3	8
Ka-Me					
Soba Shin Shu Japanese Buckwheat	2 oz	200	40	1	9
La Choy					
Ramen Noodles Chicken as prep	1 cup	200	29	7	6
Rice	½ cup	130	21	5	2
Shofar					
No Yolks	2 oz	210	41	0	91
NUTS MIXED					
dry roasted w/ peanuts	1 oz	169	7	15	5
OCTOPUS					
steamed	3 oz	140	4	2	25

FOOD	PORTION	CALS.	CARB.	FAT	PRO.
OIL					
canola	1 tbsp	124	0	14	0
corn	1 tbsp	120	0	14	0
olive	1 tbsp	119	0	14	0
OKRA					
sliced cooked	½ cup	25	6	tr	1
OLIVES					
green	4 med	15	tr	2	tr
ripe	1 lg	5	tr	tr	tr
ONION					
fried	½ cup (7.5 oz)	176	17	11	3
raw chopped	1 tbsp	4	1	tr	tr
rings breaded & fried	8 to 9	275	31	16	4
scallions raw chopped	1 tbsp	2	tr	tr	tr
Antioch Farms					
Vidalia	1 med	60	14	0	1
Vlasic					
Lightly Spiced Cocktail Onions	1 oz	4	1	0	0
ORANGE					
california valencia	1	59	14	tr	1
california navel	1	65	16	tr	1
florida	1	69	17	tr	1
Dole					
Mandarin Segments	½ cup	70	19	tr	0
ORANGE JUICE					
canned	1 cup	104	25	tr	1
chilled	1 cup	110	25	1	2
fresh	1 cup	111	26	tr	2
frzn as prep	1 cup	112	27	tr	2
Tang					
Breakfast Crystals as prep	6 oz	86	22	0	0
ORIENTAL FOOD					
chicken teriyaki	¾ cup	399	7	27	30
chop suey w/ beef & pork	1 cup	300	13	17	26
chow mein chicken	1 cup	255	10	10	31
chow mein shrimp	1 cup	221	21	10	13
chow mein vegetable	1 serv (8 oz)	90	15	3	3
egg roll meat & shrimp	1 (4.8 oz)	320	41	12	10

FOOD	PORTION	CALS.	CARB.	FAT	PRO.
egg roll vegetable	1 (3 oz)	170	28	4	5
fried rice w/ egg	6.7 oz	395	49	20	8
oriental pepper & beef	1 serv (8 oz)	90	12	0	10
spring roll deep fried	3.5 oz	202	24	9	6
sweet & sour pork	1 serv (8 oz)	250	37	8	6
OYSTERS					
battered & fried	6 (4.9 oz)	368	40	18	13
breaded & fried	6 (4.9 oz)	368	40	18	13
steamed	1 med	41	2	1	5
stew	1 cup	278	15	18	15
Bumble Bee					
Whole Canned	½ cup (3.5 oz)	100	6	4	10
PANCAKE/WAFFLE SYRUP					
low calorie	1 tbsp	12	3	0	0
pancake syrup	1 tbsp (0.7 oz)	57	15	0	0
PANCAKES					
blueberry	1 (4 in diam)	84	11	4	2
buttermilk	1, 4 in diam (1.3 oz)	74	14	1	2
plain	1 (4 in diam)	86	11	4	2
potato	1 (4 in diam)	78	4	6	2
w/ butter & syrup	3	519	91	14	8
whole wheat	1 (4 in diam)	92	13	3	4
PAPAYA					
fresh	1	117	30	tr	2
PAPAYA JUICE					
nectar	1 cup	142	36	tr	tr
PARSLEY					
Dole					
Chopped	1 tbsp	10	1	tr	tr
PARSNIPS					
fresh sliced cooked	½ cup	63	15	tr	1
PASTA					
all shapes cooked	1 cup	197	40	tr	7
fresh made w/ egg cooked	2 oz	75	14	tr	3
fresh spinach made w/ egg cooked	2 oz	74	14	tr	3
protein-fortified cooked	1 cup	188	36	tr	9

FOOD	PORTION	CALS.	CARB.	FAT	PRO.
spinach cooked	1 cup	183	37	tr	6
whole wheat cooked	1 cup (4.9 oz)	174	37	tr	7
Contadina					
Light Ravioli Cheese	1 cup (3.1 oz)	240	35	5	13
Light Ravioli Garden Vegetable	1¼ cup (3.8 oz)	290	43	6	15
Light Tortellini Garlic & Cheese	1 cup (3.6 oz)	280	50	5	15
Ravioli Beef And Garlic	1¼ cup (4 oz)	350	39	14	17
Tortellini Chicken And Vegetable	¾ cup (2.9 oz)	260	39	7	10
Di Giorno					
Ravioli Italian Herb Cheese	1 cup (3.8 oz)	350	44	13	15
Tortellini Mushroom	1 cup (3.4 oz)	290	42	7	14
Herb's					
Rotini Mixed Vegetable	2 oz	210	42	1	7

PASTA DINNERS

FOOD	PORTION	CALS.	CARB.	FAT	PRO.
lasagna	1 piece (2.5 in x 2.5 in)	374	25	21	22
manicotti	¾ cup (6.4 oz)	273	28	12	14
rigatoni w/ sausage sauce	¾ cup	260	28	12	10
spaghetti w/ meatballs & cheese	1 cup	407	38	19	21
Chef Boyardee					
ABC's & 1,2,3's In Cheese Flavor Sauce	7.5 oz	180	37	1	5
ABC's & 1,2,3's w/ Mini Meatballs	7.5 oz	260	32	11	7
Beef Ravioli	7.5 oz	190	31	4	7
Beefaroni	7.5 oz	220	31	7	7
Franco-American					
Spaghetti In Tomato Sauce w/ Cheese	½ can (7⅜ oz)	180	36	2	5
Kid's Kitchen					
Spaghetti Rings & Franks	1 cup (7.5 oz)	230	36	6	9
Kraft					
Macaroni & Cheese Deluxe Original	1 cup (6.1 oz)	320	44	10	14
Lunch Bucket					
Spaghetti'n Meatsauce	1 pkg (7.5 oz)	240	39	5	9
Micro Cup Meals					
Lasagna	1 cup (7.5 oz)	230	34	7	9
Macaroni & Cheese	1 cup (7.5 oz)	260	30	11	11

FOOD	PORTION	CALS.	CARB.	FAT	PRO.
Velveeta					
Shells & Cheese Original	1 cup (6.6 oz)	360	44	13	16
PASTA SALAD					
elbow macaroni salad	3.5 oz	160	26	5	3
pasta salad w/ vegetables	3.5 oz	140	21	4	4
PATE					
goose liver smoked	1 tbsp (13 g)	60	1	6	1
PEACH					
fresh	1	37	10	tr	1
halves dried	10	311	80	1	5
halves juice pack	1 half	34	9	tr	tr
S&W					
Whole Yellow Cling Spiced In Heavy Syrup	½ cup	90	23	0	0
PEACH JUICE					
nectar	1 cup	134	35	tr	1
PEANUT BUTTER					
chunky	2 tbsp	188	7	16	8
smooth	2 tbsp	188	7	16	8
Skippy					
Creamy w/ 2 slices white bread	1 sandwich	340	33	19	14
Tree Of Life					
Crunchy Organic No Salt	2 tbsp (1 oz)	190	7	16	8
PEANUTS					
chocolate coated	10 (1.4 oz)	208	20	13	5
dry roasted	1 oz	164	6	14	7
oil roasted	1 oz	163	5	14	7
Planters					
Honey Roasted	1 oz	160	8	13	6
PEAR					
asian	1 (4.3 oz)	51	13	tr	1
halves	10	459	122	1	3
halves in light syrup	1 half	45	12	tr	tr
pear	1	98	25	1	1
PEAR JUICE					
nectar	1 cup	149	39	tr	tr

FOOD	PORTION	CALS.	CARB.	FAT	PRO.
PEAS					
green	½ cup	59	11	tr	4
pea & potato curry	1 serv (7 oz)	284	19	22	5
split peas cooked	1 cup	231	41	1	16
Birds Eye					
Sugar Snap Deluxe	½ cup	45	9	0	2
Chun King					
Snow Pea Pods	½ pkg (3 oz)	35	4	2	2
S&W					
Petit Pois	½ cup	70	12	0	4
PECANS					
dry roasted	1 oz	187	6	18	2
PEPPERS					
chili green hot canned	1 (2.6 oz)	18	4	tr	1
chili green hot raw	1	18	4	tr	1
green cooked	1 (2.6 oz)	20	5	tr	1
jalapeno chopped canned	½ cup	17	3	tr	1
red raw	1 (2.6 oz)	20	5	tr	1
yellow raw	1 (6.5 oz)	50	12	tr	2
Hebrew National					
Hot Cherry	⅓ pepper (1 oz)	11	2	0	0
PERCH					
cooked	3 oz	99	0	1	21
PERSIMMONS					
fresh	1	32	8	tr	tr
PICKLES					
dill	1 (2.3 oz)	12	3	tr	tr
kosher dill	1 (2.3 oz)	12	3	tr	tr
quick sour	1 (1.2 oz)	4	1	tr	tr
sweet gherkin	1 sm (0.5 oz)	20	5	tr	tr
Vlasic					
Bread & Butter Chips	1 oz	30	7	0	0
PIE					
apple	⅛ of 9 in pie (5.4 oz)	411	58	19	4
blueberry	⅛ of 9 in pie (5.2 oz)	360	49	18	4

FOOD	PORTION	CALS.	CARB.	FAT	PRO.
cherry	⅛ of 9 in pie (6.3 oz)	486	69	22	5
coconut creme	⅛ of 9 in pie (4.7 oz)	396	46	21	6
custard	⅛ of 9 in pie (4.5 oz)	262	34	11	7
lemon meringue	⅛ of 9 in pie (4.5 oz)	362	50	16	5
pecan	⅛ of 9 in pie (4.3 oz)	502	64	27	6
pumpkin	⅛ of 9 in pie (5.4 oz)	316	41	14	7
PIEROGI					
pierogi	¾ cup (4.4 oz)	307	24	19	11
PIGEON PEAS					
dried cooked	½ cup	102	20	tr	6
PIKE					
cooked	3 oz	96	0	1	21
PIMIENTOS					
canned	1 tbsp	3	1	tr	tr
PINE NUTS					
pignolia dried	1 tbsp	51	1	5	2
PINEAPPLE					
fresh slice	1 slice	42	10	tr	tr
slices in light syrup	1 slice	30	8	tr	tr
Sonoma					
Pieces Dried	2 pieces (1.4 oz)	140	30	2	0
PINEAPPLE JUICE					
canned	1 cup	139	34	tr	1
PINK BEANS					
cooked	1 cup	252	47	1	15
PINTO BEANS					
Eden					
Organic	½ cup (4.4 oz)	90	17	1	5
PISTACHIOS					
dry roasted	1 oz	172	8	15	4

FOOD	PORTION	CALS.	CARB.	FAT	PRO.
PIZZA					
Boboli					
Shell + Sauce	⅛ lg shell (2.6 oz)	170	28	3	7
Celeste					
Italian Bread Deluxe	1 (5.1 oz)	290	36	11	16
Italian Bread Garlic & Herb Zesty Chicken	1 (5 oz)	260	34	8	17
Empire					
Bagel	1 (2 oz)	150	15	5	7
Healthy Choice					
French Bread Cheese	1 (5.6 oz)	310	49	4	20
Jeno's					
Pizza Rolls Cheese	6	240	23	12	8
Kid Cuisine					
Hamburger	1 (8.30 oz)	400	61	11	14
MicroMagic					
Deep Dish Combination	1 (6.5 oz)	605	60	34	14
Mrs. P's					
Pepperoni	½ pizza	250	26	13	8
Pappalo's					
Pan Combination	⅙ pizza	340	34	15	17
Pepperidge Farm					
Croissant Pastry Deluxe	1	440	43	23	16
Pillsbury					
Microwave Sausage	½ pizza	280	29	13	13
Special Delivery					
Organic	⅓ pizza (5.3 oz)	320	46	9	13
Stouffer's					
Lunch Express Double Cheese	1 pkg (5.9 oz)	420	41	19	21
Tombstone					
12 in Cheese Sausage & Mushroom	⅕ pie (4.5 oz)	320	29	16	15
For One ½ Less Fat Vegetable	1 pie (7.2 oz)	360	46	10	22
Totino's					
Party Hamburger	½ pizza	370	35	19	15
Weight Watchers					
Cheese	1 (6.03 oz)	300	36	7	24

FOOD	PORTION	CALS.	CARB.	FAT	PRO.
PLANTAINS					
sliced cooked	½ cup	89	24	tr	1
PLUMS					
fresh	1	36	9	tr	1
purple in heavy syrup	3	119	31	tr	tr
POLLACK					
baked	3 oz	100	0	1	21
POMEGRANATES					
pomegranate	1	104	26	tr	1
POMPANO					
florida cooked	3 oz	179	0	10	20
POPCORN					
air-popped	1 cup (0.3 oz)	31	6	tr	1
caramel coated	1 cup (1.2 oz)	152	28	5	1
oil popped	1 cup (0.4 oz)	55	6	3	1
Orville Redenbacher's					
Microwave Gourmet Light	3 cups	70	8	3	2
POPCORN CAKES					
Lundberg					
Organic Lightly Salted	1	60	12	1	1
Mother's					
Unsalted	1 (0.3 oz)	35	7	0	1
Quaker					
White Cheddar	1 (0.4 oz)	40	8	0	1
PORK					
center loin chop, broiled	1 (3.1 oz)	275	0	24	24
center loin, roasted	3 oz	259	0	18	22
loin w/ fat, roasted	3 oz	271	0	21	20
pork roast	2 oz	70	0	3	10
spareribs, braised	3 oz	338	0	26	26
tenderloin lean only roasted	3 oz	141	0	4	24
POT PIE					
beef	⅓ pie 9 in (7.4 oz)	515	39	30	21
chicken	⅓ pie 9 in (8.1 oz)	545	42	31	23
POTATO					
baked topped w/ cheese sauce	1	475	47	29	15
baked topped w/ cheese sauce & bacon	1	451	44	26	18

FOOD	PORTION	CALS.	CARB.	FAT	PRO.
baked topped w/ cheese sauce & broccoli	1	402	47	14	14
baked topped w/ cheese sauce & chili	1	481	56	22	23
baked topped w/ sour cream & chives	1	394	50	22	7
baked w/ skin	1 (6.5 oz)	220	51	tr	5
boiled	½ cup	68	16	tr	1
canned	½ cup	54	12	tr	1
french fries	10 strips	111	17	4	2
hashed brown	½ cup	170	22	9	2
instant mashed flakes as prep w/ whole milk & butter	½ cup	118	16	6	2
mashed	½ cup	111	18	4	2
potato dumpling	3½ oz	334	74	1	7
potato pancakes	1 (1.3 oz)	101	11	7	2
potato puffs	½ cup	138	19	7	2
potato salad	½ cup	179	14	10	3
scalloped	½ cup	105	13	5	4
POUT					
ocean baked	3 oz	86	0	1	18
PRETZELS					
chocolate covered	1 (0.4 oz)	50	8	2	1
rods	4 (2 oz)	229	48	2	6
sticks	10	10	2	tr	tr
twist	1 (0.5 oz)	65	13	1	2
whole wheat	2 sm (1 oz)	103	23	1	3
J&J					
Soft	1 (2.25 oz)	170	37	0	6
PRUNE JUICE					
canned	1 cup	181	45	tr	2
PRUNES					
Del Monte					
Unpitted Dried	⅓ cup (1.4 oz)	110	12	0	1
PUDDING					
bread pudding	½ cup (4.4 oz)	212	31	7	7
chocolate ready-to-use	1 pkg (5 oz)	189	32	6	4
lemon ready-to-use	1 pkg (5 oz)	177	36	4	tr

FOOD	PORTION	CALS.	CARB.	FAT	PRO.
rice	½ cup (5.3 oz)	217	40	4	6
tapioca	½ cup (5 oz)	147	28	2	4
vanilla ready-to-use	1 pkg (4 oz)	146	25	4	3
PUDDING POPS					
chocolate	1 (1.6 oz)	72	12	2	2
vanilla	1 (1.6 oz)	75	13	2	2
PUMMELO					
fresh	1	228	59	tr	5
PUMPKIN					
seeds salted & roasted	1 oz	148	4	12	9
QUICHE					
cheese	1 slice (3 oz)	283	16	20	11
lorraine	1 slice (3 oz)	352	18	25	15
mushroom	1 slice (3 oz)	256	17	18	9
QUINOA					
quinoa	½ cup	318	59	5	11
RABBIT					
domestic w/o bone roasted	3 oz	167	0	7	25
RACCOON					
roasted	3 oz	217	0	12	25
RADICCHIO					
raw shredded	½ cup	5	1	tr	tr
RADISHES					
daikon raw sliced	½ cup	8	2	tr	tr
red raw	10	7	2	tr	tr
RAISINS					
chocolate coated	10 (0.4 oz)	39	7	2	tr
seedless	1 tbsp	27	7	tr	tr
Del Monte					
Yogurt Raisins Vanilla	1 pkg (1 oz)	120	22	3	2
RASPBERRIES					
fresh	1 cup	61	14	1	1
RED BEANS					
Allen					
Canned	½ cup (4.5 oz)	160	19	1	6

FOOD	PORTION	CALS.	CARB.	FAT	PRO.
RELISH					
hamburger	1 tbsp	19	5	tr	tr
hot dog	1 tbsp	14	4	tr	tr
RHUBARB					
as prep w/ sugar	½ cup	139	37	tr	tr
RICE					
brown long-grain cooked	½ cup	109	23	tr	3
pilaf	½ cup	84	11	3	4
risotto	6.6 oz	426	65	18	6
spanish	¾ cup	363	19	27	11
white long-grain cooked	½ cup	131	28	tr	3
white long-grain instant cooked	½ cup	80	17	tr	2
Casbah					
Basmati as prep	1 cup	158	36	tr	3
Rice-A-Roni					
Beef	½ cup	140	24	4	4
Superfino					
Arborio Rice	½ cup	100	22	0	2
RICE CAKES					
Hain					
Mini Barbeque	½ oz	70	10	3	1
Ka-Me					
Sesame	16 pieces (1 oz)	120	24	2	3
Lundberg					
Organic Lightly Salted	1	60	14	1	1
Mother's					
Mini Caramel	5 (0.5 oz)	50	12	0	1
Quaker					
Salted	1 (0.3 oz)	35	7	0	1
ROCKFISH					
pacific cooked	1 fillet (5.2 oz)	180	0	3	36
ROLL					
brown & serve	1 (1 oz)	85	14	2	2
cheese	1 (2.3 oz)	238	29	12	5
cinnamon raisin	1 (2¾ in)	223	31	10	4
dinner	1 (1 oz)	85	14	2	2
egg	1 (2½ in)	107	18	2	3
french	1 (1.3 oz)	105	19	2	3

FOOD	PORTION	CALS.	CARB.	FAT	PRO.
hamburger	1 (1½ oz)	123	22	2	4
hard	1 (3½ in)	167	30	2	6
hot cross bun	1	202	38	4	5
hotdog	1 (1½ oz)	123	22	2	4
kaiser	1 (3½ in)	167	30	2	6
rye	1 (1 oz)	81	15	1	3
submarine	1 (4.7 oz)	155	30	2	5
whole wheat	1 (1 oz)	75	15	1	3

ROUGHY

FOOD	PORTION	CALS.	CARB.	FAT	PRO.
orange baked	3 oz	75	0	1	16

SABLEFISH

FOOD	PORTION	CALS.	CARB.	FAT	PRO.
smoked	1 oz	72	0	6	5

SALAD

FOOD	PORTION	CALS.	CARB.	FAT	PRO.
chef w/o dressing	1½ cups	386	9	28	24
tossed w/o dressing	1½ cups	32	7	tr	3
tossed w/o dressing w/ cheese & egg	1½ cups	102	5	6	9
tossed w/o dressing w/ chicken	1½ cups	105	4	2	17
tossed w/o dressing w/ pasta & seafood	1½ cups (14.6 oz)	380	32	21	16
tossed w/o dressing w/ shrimp	1½ cups	107	7	2	15
waldorf	½ cup	79	6	6	1

SALAD DRESSING

FOOD	PORTION	CALS.	CARB.	FAT	PRO.
french	1 tbsp	67	3	6	tr
french reduced calorie	1 tbsp	22	4	1	0
italian	1 tbsp	69	2	7	tr
italian reduced calorie	1 tbsp	16	1	2	tr
russian	1 tbsp	76	2	8	tr
russian reduced calorie	1 tbsp	23	5	1	tr
thousand island	1 tbsp	59	2	6	tr
thousand island reduced calorie	1 tbsp	24	3	2	tr
Kraft					
Free Blue Cheese	2 tbsp (1.2 oz)	50	12	0	tr
Free French	2 tbsp (1.2 oz)	50	12	0	0
Free Italian	2 tbsp (1.1 oz)	10	2	0	0
Free Ranch	1 tbsp (1.2 oz)	50	11	0	tr
Free Red Wine Vinegar	2 tbsp (1.1 oz)	15	3	0	0
Free Thousand Island	2 tbsp (1.2 oz)	45	11	0	0

FOOD	PORTION	CALS.	CARB.	FAT	PRO.
Marzetti					
Fat Free Slaw	2 tbsp	45	11	0	0
Newman's Own					
Italian Light	1 tbsp (0.5 fl oz)	10	tr	tr	tr
Walden Farms					
Fat Free Balsamic Vinaigrette	2 tbsp (1 oz)	15	3	0	0
Fat Free Caesar	2 tbsp (1 oz)	25	4	0	1
SALMON					
baked	3 oz	155	0	7	22
pink w/ bone canned	3 oz	118	0	5	17
salmon cake	1 (3 oz)	241	6	15	18
smoked	1 oz	33	0	1	5
SALSA					
Chi-Chi's					
Hot	2 tbsp (1 oz)	10	1	0	0
Frito Lay					
Medium	1 oz	12	2	0	0
Muir Glen					
Organic Fat Free Mild	2 tbsp (1.1 oz)	10	2	0	tr
Newman's Own					
Bandito Hot	1 tbsp (0.7 oz)	6	tr	tr	tr
Old El Paso					
Thick'n Chunky Green Chili	2 tbsp	3	1	0	0
SAPODILLA					
fresh	1	140	34	2	1
SARDINES					
in oil w/ bone canned	2	50	0	3	6
in tomato sauce w/ bone canned	1	68	0	5	6
Port Clyde					
In Mustard Sauce	1 can (3.75 oz)	150	1	9	18
Underwood					
Brisling In Olive Oil	3.75 oz	260	1	20	19
SAUCE					
cheese as prep w/ milk	1 cup	307	23	17	16
teriyaki	1 oz	30	6	0	2
Cheez Whiz					
Zap-A-Pack	2 tbsp (1.2 oz)	90	3	8	3

FOOD	PORTION	CALS.	CARB.	FAT	PRO.
Golden Dipt					
Seafood Cocktail	1 tbsp	20	5	0	0
Hellman's					
Tartar	1 tbsp (14 g)	70	tr	8	tr
Ka-Me					
Duck Sauce	2 tbsp (1 oz)	80	20	0	0
Knorr					
Hollandaise as prep	2 oz	170	5	18	2
Lea & Perrins					
Worcestershire	1 tsp	5	1	tr	tr
McIlhenny					
Tabasco	1 tsp	1	tr	tr	tr
Old El Paso					
Picante Thick'n Chunky Hot	2 tbsp	10	2	0	0
Progresso					
Alfredo	½ cup	340	6	30	13
SAUERKRAUT					
canned	½ cup	22	5	tr	1
SAUERKRAUT JUICE					
S&W					
Juice	4 oz	14	3	0	1
SAUSAGE					
bratwurst pork cooked	1 link (3 oz)	256	2	22	12
italian pork cooked	1 (2.4 oz)	216	1	17	13
kielbasa pork	1 oz	88	1	8	8
knockwurst pork & beef	1 oz	87	1	8	3
smoked pork	1 link (2.4 oz)	265	1	22	15
vienna canned	1 (0.5 oz)	45	tr	4	2
zungenwurst (tongue)	3.5 oz	285	0	24	17
Aidells					
Andouille Cajun Cooked	1 (3.5 oz)	220	1	17	16
Lemon Chicken Cooked	1 (3.5 oz)	220	1	16	15
Healthy Choice					
Low Fat Smoked	2 oz	70	4	2	8
Low Fat Smoked Polska Kielbasa	2 oz	70	4	2	8
Hillshire					
Links 80% Fat Free Smokies	2 oz	130	2	10	8

FOOD	PORTION	CALS.	CARB.	FAT	PRO.
Hormel					
Light & Lean 97 Dinner Smoked	2 oz	60	2	2	8
Jimmy Dean					
Pattie Pre-Cooked	1 (1.9 oz)	230	0	22	7
Jones					
Brown & Serve Beef	1	90	tr	9	3
Brown & Serve Light	1	60	1	5	3
Scrapple	1 slice	90	5	6	4
Louis Rich					
Turkey	2.5 oz	110	3	6	11
Old Smokehouse					
Summer Sausage	1 oz	110	1	10	4
Oscar Mayer					
Pork Cooked	2 links (1.7 oz)	170	1	15	9
Perdue					
Hot Italian Turkey cooked	1 (2 oz)	94	0	6	10
Shofar					
Knockwurst Beef	1 (3 oz)	260	tr	23	11

SAUSAGE DISHES

sausage roll	1 (2.3 oz)	311	22	24	5

SAUSAGE SUBSTITUTES

Lightlife					
Lean Links Italian	1.5 oz	83	5	3	5
Morningstar Farms					
Breakfast Patties	2 (76 g)	190	7	12	15
Worthington					
Veja-Links	2 (62 g)	140	4	10	8

SCALLOP

breaded & fried	2 lg	67	3	3	6

SCONE

fruit	1 (1.75 oz)	158	27	5	4
plain	1 (1.75 oz)	181	27	7	4

SCROD

Gorton's					
Microwave Entree Baked	1 pkg	320	18	18	17

SCUP

fresh baked	3 oz	115	0	3	21

FOOD	PORTION	CALS.	CARB.	FAT	PRO.
SEAWEED					
Eden					
Kombu	3.5 in piece (3.3 g)	10	2	0	0
Nori	1 sheet (2.5 g)	10	1	0	1
Sushi Nori	1 sheet (2.5 g)	10	1	0	1
Maine Coast					
Dulse	⅓ cup (7 g)	18	3	0	2
Kelp	⅓ cup (7 g)	17	3	0	1
Laver	⅓ cup (7 g)	22	3	0	2
SESAME					
sesame crunch candy	20 pieces (1.2 oz)	181	18	12	4
Arrowhead					
Sesame Tahini	1 oz	170	4	17	6
SHAD					
baked	3 oz	214	0	15	18
roe baked w/ butter & lemon	3.5 oz	126	2	3	22
SHALLOTS					
raw chopped	1 tbsp	7	2	tr	tr
SHARK					
batter-dipped & fried	3 oz	194	5	12	16
SHEEPSHEAD FISH					
cooked	3 oz	107	0	1	22
SHELLFISH SUBSTITUTES					
surimi	3 oz	84	6	1	13
SHELLIE BEANS					
canned	½ cup	37	8	tr	2
SHERBET					
orange	½ cup (4 fl oz)	132	29	2	1
SHRIMP					
breaded & fried	4 large	73	3	4	6
canned	3 oz	102	1	2	20
cooked	4 large	22	0	tr	5
jambalaya	¾ cup	188	26	5	11
SMELT					
rainbow cooked	3 oz	106	0	3	19

FOOD	PORTION	CALS.	CARB.	FAT	PRO.
SNACKS					
oriental mix	1 oz	155	9	12	6
pork skins	½ oz	77	0	4	9
Chex					
Snack Mix Traditional	⅔ cup (1.2 oz)	150	23	5	3
Combos					
Cheddar Cheese Cracker	1 pkg (1.7 oz)	250	28	13	5
Cornnuts					
Original	1 oz	120	22	4	2
Energy Food Factory					
Poprice Cheddar Cheese	½ oz	60	8	3	2
Hapi					
Chili Bits	½ cup (1 oz)	110	25	0	3
Weight Watchers					
Cheese Curls	½ oz	70	10	2	1
SNAIL					
cooked	3 oz	233	13	1	41
SNAP BEANS					
canned	½ cup	13	3	tr	1
italian canned	½ cup	13	3	tr	1
yellow canned	½ cup	13	3	tr	1
SNAPPER					
cooked	3 oz	109	0	1	22
SODA					
club	12 oz	0	0	0	0
cola	12 oz	151	39	tr	tr
cream	12 oz	191	49	0	0
diet cola	12 oz	2	tr	0	tr
ginger ale	12 oz can	124	32	0	tr
grape	12 oz	161	42	0	0
lemon lime	12 oz	149	38	0	0
root beer	12 oz	152	39	0	tr
Canada Dry					
Seltzer Strawberry	8 fl oz	0	0	0	0
Orangina					
Sparkling Citrus	6 fl oz	80	19	0	0
Yoo-Hoo					
Original	9 fl oz	150	31	tr	3

FOOD	PORTION	CALS.	CARB.	FAT	PRO.
SOLE					
battered & fried	3.2 oz	211	15	11	13
breaded & fried	3.2 oz	211	15	11	13
cooked	3 oz	99	0	1	21
SOUFFLE					
cheese	3.5 oz	253	10	20	11
spinach	1 cup	218	3	18	11
SOUP					
asparagus cream of as prep w/ milk	1 cup	161	16	8	6
beef broth ready-to-serve	1 cup	16	tr	1	3
beef noodle as prep w/water	1 cup	84	9	3	5
beef stew soup	1 cup (8.8 oz)	221	20	5	23
black bean turtle soup	1 cup	218	40	1	14
celery cream of as prep w/ milk	1 cup	165	15	10	6
cheese as prep w/ milk	1 cup	230	16	15	9
chicken broth as prep w/ water	1 cup	39	1	1	5
chicken cream of as prep w/ water	1 cup	116	9	7	3
chicken gumbo as prep w/water	1 cup	56	8	1	3
chicken noodle as prep w/ water	1 cup	75	9	2	4
chicken rice as prep w/ water	1 cup	251	7	2	4
clam chowder manhattan as prep w/ water	1 cup	77	12	2	2
clam chowder new england as prep w/ milk	1 cup	163	17	7	9
corn & cheese chowder	¾ cup	215	21	12	9
escarole ready-to-serve	1 cup	27	2	2	2
french onion as prep w/ water	1 cup	57	8	2	4
gazpacho ready-to-serve	1 cup	57	1	2	9
greek	¾ cup	63	7	2	4
hot & sour	1 serv (14 oz)	173	8	8	15
minestrone as prep w/water	1 cup	83	11	3	4
mushroom cream of as prep w/ water	1 cup	129	9	9	2
oxtail	5 oz	64	7	3	4
oyster stew as prep w/ milk	1 cup	134	10	8	6
pasta e fagioli	1 cup (8.8 oz)	194	30	5	9
pepperpot as prep w/ water	1 cup	103	9	5	6
potato cream of as prep w/ milk	1 cup	148	17	6	6

FOOD	PORTION	CALS.	CARB.	FAT	PRO.
scotch broth as prep w/ water	1 cup	80	9	3	5
split pea w/ ham as prep w/ water	1 cup	189	28	4	10
tomato as prep w/ milk	1 cup	160	22	6	6
vegetarian vegetable as prep w/ water	1 cup	72	12	2	2
vichyssoise	1 cup	148	17	6	6

SOUR CREAM

sour cream	1 tbsp	26	1	3	tr
Breakstone					
Free	2 tbsp (1.1 oz)	35	6	0	2
Half & Half	2 tbsp (1.1 oz)	45	2	4	1

SOUR CREAM SUBSTITUTES

nondairy	1 oz	59	2	6	1

SOY

lecithin	1 tbsp	104	0	14	0
soy milk	1 cup	79	4	5	7
soya cheese	1.4 oz	128	tr	11	7

SOY SAUCE

shoyu	1 tbsp	9	2	tr	1
soy sauce	1 tbsp	7	1	tr	tr
tamari	1 tbsp	11	1	tr	2
Kikkoman					
Lite	1 tbsp	13	2	0	1

SOYBEANS

dried cooked	1 cup	298	17	15	29
dry-roasted	½ cup	387	28	19	34
sprouts raw	½ cup	43	3	2	5
sprouts stir fried	1 cup	125	9	7	13

SPAGHETTI SAUCE

marinara sauce	1 cup	171	25	8	4
spaghetti sauce	1 cup	272	40	12	12
Classico					
Spicy Red Pepper	4 fl oz	50	6	2	2
Contadina					
Alfredo	½ cup (4.2 fl oz)	400	8	38	7
Light Alfredo	½ cup (4.2 fl oz)	190	10	13	8
Pesto With Sun Dried Tomatoes	¼ cup (2 oz)	250	6	24	3

FOOD	PORTION	CALS.	CARB.	FAT	PRO.
Del Monte					
With Meat	½ cup (4.4 oz)	40	13	2	3
Mama Rizzo's					
Primavera Vegetable	½ cup (4.2 oz)	50	8	2	2
Muir Glen					
Organic Fat Free Tomato Basil	½ cup (4.3 oz)	50	10	0	2
Progresso					
Bolognese	½ cup	150	12	12	10
SPANISH FOOD					
burrito w/ beans	2 (7.6 oz)	448	71	14	14
burrito w/ beans & cheese	2 (6.5 oz)	377	55	12	15
burrito w/ beans & chili peppers	2 (7.2 oz)	413	58	15	16
burrito w/ beans & meat	2 (8.1 oz)	508	66	18	22
burrito w/ beans cheese & beef	2 (7.1 oz)	331	40	13	15
burrito w/ beans cheese & chili peppers	2 (11.8 oz)	663	85	23	33
burrito w/ beef	2 (7.7 oz)	523	59	21	27
burrito w/ beef & chili peppers	2 (7.1 oz)	426	49	17	22
burrito w/ beef cheese & chili peppers	2 (10.7 oz)	634	64	25	41
chimichanga w/ beef	1 (6.1 oz)	425	43	20	20
chimichanga w/ beef & cheese	1 (6.4 oz)	443	39	23	20
chimichanga w/ beef & red chili peppers	1 (6.7 oz)	424	46	19	18
chimichanga w/ beef cheese & red chili peppers	1 (6.3 oz)	364	38	18	15
enchilada w/ cheese	1 (5.7 oz)	320	29	19	10
enchilada w/ cheese & beef	1 (6.7 oz)	324	30	18	12
enchirito w/ cheese beef & beans	1 (6.8 oz)	344	34	16	18
frijoles w/ cheese	1 cup (5.9 oz)	226	29	8	11
nachos w/ cheese	6 to 8 (4 oz)	345	36	19	9
nachos w/ cheese & jalapeno peppers	6 to 8 (7.2 oz)	607	60	34	17
nachos w/ cheese beans ground beef & peppers	6 to 8 (8.9 oz)	568	56	31	20
nachos w/ cinnamon & sugar	6 to 8 (3.8 oz)	592	63	36	7
taco	1 sm (6 oz)	370	27	21	21
taco salad	1½ cups	279	24	15	13

FOOD	PORTION	CALS.	CARB.	FAT	PRO.
taco salad w/ chili con carne	1½ cups	288	27	13	17
tostada w/ beans & cheese	1 (5.1 oz)	223	27	10	10
tostada w/ beans beef & cheese	1 (7.9 oz)	334	30	17	16
tostada w/ beef & cheese	1 (5.7 oz)	315	23	16	19
tostada w/ guacamole	2 (9.2 oz)	360	32	23	12
SPINACH					
cooked	½ cup	21	3	tr	3
raw chopped	½ cup	6	1	tr	1
Stouffer's					
Creamed	½ cup (2.25 oz)	150	8	12	4
SPINACH JUICE					
juice	3½ oz	7	1	0	1
SPORTS DRINKS					
Gatorade					
All Flavors	1 cup (8 oz)	50	14	0	0
PowerAde					
All Flavors	8 fl oz	72	19	0	0
Slice					
All Sport Diet Lemon Lime	8 fl oz	1	0	0	tr
All Sport Lemon Lime	8 fl oz	72	19	0	tr
Snapple					
Sport Orange	1 bottle	80	20	0	0
SQUASH					
acorn cubed baked	½ cup	57	15	tr	1
butternut baked	½ cup	41	11	tr	1
crookneck sliced cooked	½ cup	18	4	tr	1
hubbard cooked mashed	½ cup	35	8	tr	2
scallop sliced cooked	½ cup	14	3	tr	1
spaghetti cooked	½ cup	23	5	tr	1
SQUID					
fried	3 oz	149	7	6	15
STAR FRUIT					
Sonoma					
Dried	7-9 pieces (1.4 oz)	140	34	0	1
STRAWBERRIES					
fresh	1 cup	45	10	1	1

FOOD	PORTION	CALS.	CARB.	FAT	PRO.
STRAWBERRY JUICE					
Kern's					
Nectar	6 fl oz	110	28	0	0
STUFFING/DRESSING					
bread dry as prep	½ cup	178	22	9	3
cornbread as prep	½ cup	179	22	9	3
sausage	½ cup	292	40	11	8
STURGEON					
smoked	1 oz	48	0	1	9
SUGAR					
white	1 packet (6 g)	25	6	0	0
SUGAR SUBSTITUTES					
Equal					
Packet	1 pkg	4	tr	0	0
Weight Watchers					
Sweet'nėr	1 pkg	4	1	0	0
SUNFLOWER					
dry roasted salted	1 oz	165	7	14	5
Planters					
Kernels Salted	1 oz	170	4	14	7
SUSHI					
california roll	1 piece (0.8 oz)	28	4	1	1
kim chi	⅓ cup (5.8 oz)	18	4	tr	1
sashimi	1 serving (6 oz)	198	4	7	24
tuna roll	1 piece (0.7 oz)	23	3	tr	2
vegetable roll	1 piece (1.2 oz)	27	5	1	1
vinegared ginger	⅓ cup (1.6 oz)	48	12	tr	1
wasabi	2 tsp (0.3 oz)	5	1	tr	tr
yellowtail roll	1 piece (0.6 oz)	25	3	1	1
SWEET POTATO					
baked w/ skin	1 (3½ oz)	118	28	tr	2
candied	3½ oz	144	29	3	1
canned in syrup	½ cup	106	25	tr	1
SWEETBREADS					
beef braised	3 oz	230	0	15	23
SWISS CHARD					
cooked	½ cup	18	4	tr	2

FOOD	PORTION	CALS.	CARB.	FAT	PRO.
SWORDFISH					
cooked	3 oz	132	0	4	22
SYRUP					
Eden					
Barley Malt Organic Syrup	1 tbsp (0.7 fl oz)	60	14	0	1
Smucker's					
All Flavors Fruit Syrup	2 tbsp	100	26	0	0
Tree Of Life					
Maple	¼ cup (2.1 oz)	200	53	0	0
TAMARIND					
fresh	1	5	1	tr	tr
TANGERINE JUICE					
frzn sweetened as prep	1 cup	110	27	tr	1
TEA/HERBAL TEA					
brewed tea	6 oz	2	tr	0	0
Bigelow					
Herbal	5 fl oz	tr	tr	tr	tr
TEMPEH					
tempeh	½ cup	165	14	6	16
White Wave					
Burger	1 patty (3 oz)	110	10	3	12
TILEFISH					
cooked	½ fillet (5.3 oz)	220	0	7	37
TOFU					
firm	½ cup	183	5	11	20
fresh fried	1 piece (½ oz)	35	1	3	2
Mori-Nu					
Lite Extra Firm	1 in slice (3 oz)	35	1	1	6
Nasoya					
Silken	⅙ block (3 oz)	50	2	2	5
White Wave					
Soft	4 oz	120	1	7	12
TOMATILLO					
fresh	1 (1.2 oz)	11	2	tr	tr
TOMATO					
green	1	30	6	tr	1
red	1 (4½ oz)	26	6	tr	1

FOOD	PORTION	CALS.	CARB.	FAT	PRO.
stewed	1 cup	80	13	3	2
sun dried	1 piece	5	1	tr	tr
sun dried in oil	1 piece (3 g)	6	1	tr	tr
TOMATO JUICE					
tomato juice	6 oz	32	8	tr	1
TONGUE					
beef simmered	3 oz	241	tr	18	19
TROUT					
baked	3 oz	162	0	7	23
TRUFFLES					
fresh	3½ oz	25	17	1	6
TUNA					
canned light in oil	3 oz	169	0	7	25
canned light in water	3 oz	99	0	1	22
canned white in oil	3 oz	158	0	7	23
canned white in water	3 oz	116	0	2	23
fresh cooked	3 oz	157	0	5	25
TUNA DISHES					
tuna salad	3 oz	159	8	8	14
tuna salad submarine sandwich w/ lettuce & oil	1	584	55	28	30
Tuna Helper					
Buttery Rice as prep	⅕ pkg (6 oz)	280	32	11	13
Tuna Salad as prep	⅕ pkg (5.5 oz)	420	29	27	14
TURBOT					
european baked	3 oz	104	0	3	17
TURKEY					
bologna	1 oz	57	tr	4	4
breast	1 slice (¾ oz)	23	0	tr	5
breast w/ skin roasted	4 oz	212	0	8	32
canned w/ broth	½ can (2.5 oz)	116	0	5	17
ground cooked	3 oz	188	0	11	20
leg w/ skin roasted	2.5 oz	147	0	7	20
pastrami	2 oz	80	1	4	10
patties battered & fried	1 (3.3 oz)	266	15	17	13
poultry salad sandwich spread	1 tbsp	109	1	2	2
salami cooked	1 pkg (8 oz)	446	1	31	37

FOOD	PORTION	CALS.	CARB.	FAT	PRO.
turkey sticks battered & fried	1 stick (2.3 oz)	178	11	11	9
wing w/ skin roasted	1 (6.5 oz)	426	0	23	51
Alpine Lace					
Breast Fat Free	2 oz	50	0	0	12
Empire					
Patties	1 (3.1 oz)	200	14	10	13
Healthy Choice					
Deli-Thin Honey Roast & Smoked	6 slices (2 oz)	70	2	2	10
Hillshire					
Lunch 'N Munch Smoked Turkey/ Cheddar/ Brownie	1 pkg (4.5 oz)	400	34	22	17
Hormel					
Light & Lean 97 Breast Sliced	1 slice (1 oz)	30	0	1	5
Louis Rich					
Deli-Thin Smoked Breast	4 slices (1.8 oz)	50	1	1	9
Skinless Hickory Smoked Breast	2 oz	60	1	1	12
Oscar Mayer					
Free Smoked Breast	4 slices (1.8 oz)	40	2	0	8
Lunchables Fun Pack Turkey/ Surger Cooler	1 pkg (11.2 oz)	440	60	16	14
Wampler Longacre					
Burger Barbecue	1 (4 oz)	240	4	17	19

TURKEY DISHES

gravy & turkey	1 cup (8.4 oz)	160	11	6	14

TURKEY SUBSTITUTES

Worthington					
Smoked Turkey Slices	4 slices (76 g)	180	5	12	13

TURNIPS

cooked mashed	½ cup (4.2 oz)	47	10	tr	2
greens	½ cup	17	3	tr	2

VEAL

cutlet lean only braised	3 oz	172	0	4	31
cutlet lean only fried	3 oz	156	0	4	28
ground broiled	3 oz	146	0	6	21
loin chop w/ bone lean & fat braised	1 chop (2.8 oz)	227	0	14	24

VEAL DISHES

parmigiana	4.2 oz	279	6	18	22

FOOD	PORTION	CALS.	CARB.	FAT	PRO.
VEGETABLE JUICE					
V8					
Original	6 fl oz	35	8	0	1
VEGETABLES MIXED					
pakoras	1 (2 oz)	108	12	5	5
ratatouille	8.8 oz	190	10	16	2
samosa	2 (4 oz)	519	25	46	3
succotash	½ cup	111	23	1	5
VENISON					
roasted	3 oz	134	0	3	26
VINEGAR					
cider	1 tbsp	tr	1	0	tr
Ka-Me					
Rice Wine Chinese	1 tbsp (0.5 fl oz)	5	1	0	0
White House					
Red Wine	2 tbsp	4	2	0	0
WAFFLES					
buttermilk	1, 4 in sq (1.2 oz)	88	14	3	2
plain	1, 4 in sq (1.2 oz)	88	14	3	2
WALNUTS					
english dried	1 oz	182	5	18	4
WATER CHESTNUTS					
chinese sliced canned	½ cup	35	9	tr	1
WATERCRESS					
raw chopped	½ cup	2	tr	tr	tr
WATERMELON					
wedge	1/16 melon	152	35	2	3
WAX BEANS					
Seneca					
Canned	½ cup	25	6	0	1
WHEAT					
Near East					
Taboule Salad Mix as prep	⅔ cup	120	23	3	3
White Wave					
Seitan	½ pkg (4 oz)	140	4	0	31
WHEAT GERM					
plain toasted	¼ cup	108	14	3	8

FOOD	PORTION	CALS.	CARB.	FAT	PRO.
WHIPPED TOPPINGS					
Cool Whip					
Extra Creamy	1 tbsp	13	1	1	0
Lite	1 tbsp	9	1	1	0
WHITE BEANS					
canned	1 cup	306	58	1	19
Progresso					
Cannellini	½ cup	80	19	tr	8
WHITEFISH					
smoked	1 oz	39	0	tr	7
WHITING					
cooked	3 oz	98	0	1	20
WILD RICE					
cooked	½ cup	83	18	tr	3
WINE					
madeira	3.5 oz	169	10	0	0
port	3.5 oz	156	11	0	tr
red	3½ oz	74	2	0	tr
rose	3½ oz	73	2	0	tr
sherry	2 oz	84	5	0	tr
sweet dessert	2 oz	90	7	0	tr
white	3½ oz	70	1	0	tr
YEAST					
baker's compressed	1 cake (0.6 oz)	18	3	tr	1
baker's dry	1 tbsp	35	5	1	5
brewer's dry	1 tbsp	25	3	tr	3
YELLOWTAIL					
baked	3 oz	159	0	6	25
YOGURT					
fruit lowfat	8 oz	225	42	3	9
fruit lowfat	4 oz	113	21	1	5
plain	8 oz	139	11	7	8
plain lowfat	8 oz	144	16	4	12
plain no fat	8 oz	127	17	tr	13
vanilla lowfat	8 oz	194	31	3	11
YOGURT FROZEN					
chocolate soft serve	½ cup (4 fl oz)	115	18	4	3
vanilla soft serve	½ cup (4 fl oz)	114	17	4	3

FOOD	PORTION	CALS.	CARB.	FAT	PRO.
ZUCCHINI					
fresh sliced cooked	½ cup	14	4	tr	1
italian style canned	½ cup	33	8	tr	1
raw sliced	½ cup	9	2	tr	1
Empire					
Breaded	1 (2.9 oz)	100	18	0	5